Reflexology
for Women

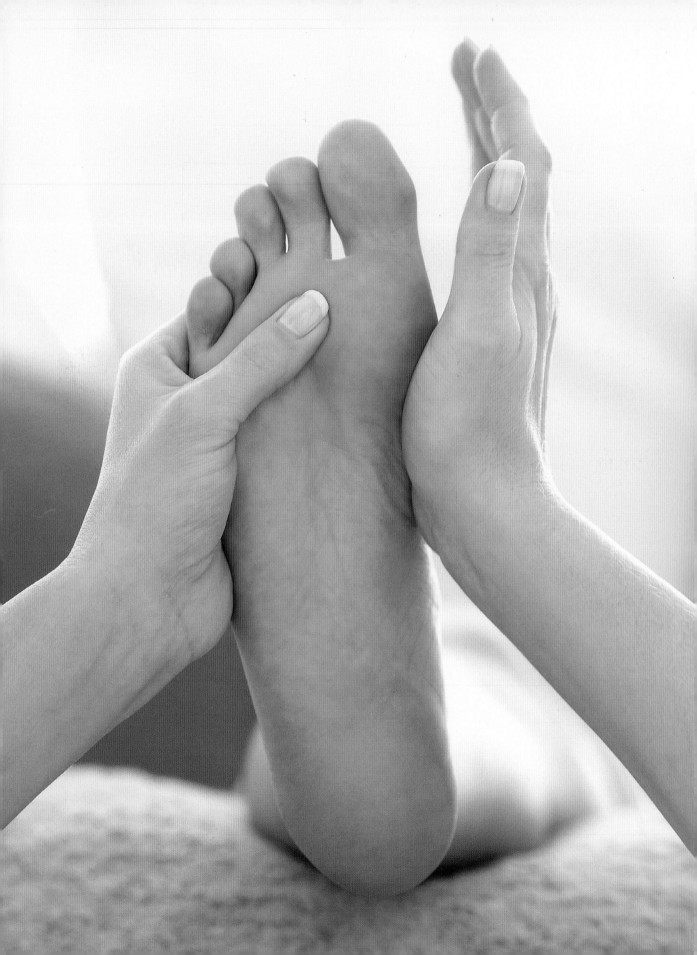

Reflexology for Women

Simple step-by-step treatments for women of all ages

Ann Gillanders

GAIA BOOKS

Reconnect with yourself
and the planet

First published in Great Britain in 2006 by
Gaia, a division of Octopus Publishing Group Ltd
2–4 Heron Quays, London E14 4JP

Ann Gillanders asserts the moral right to be identified as the author
of this work.

ISBN-13: 978-185675-228-2
ISBN-10: 1-85675-228-3

A CIP catalogue record for this book is available from the British Library.

Printed and bound in China

10 9 8 7 6 5 4 3 2 1

All reasonable care has been taken in the preparation of this book, but
the information it contains is not intended to take the place of medical
care under the direct supervision of a qualified doctor. Before making
any changes in your health regime, always consult your doctor. Always
seek advice from a professional reflexologist before treating women
during the first 14 weeks of pregnancy, particularly if they have a history
of miscarriage. Any application of the ideas and information contained
in this book is at the reader's sole discretion and risk.

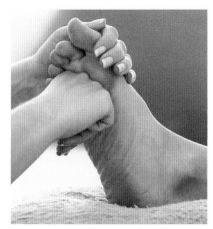
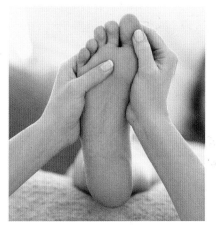
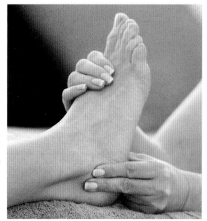

Contents

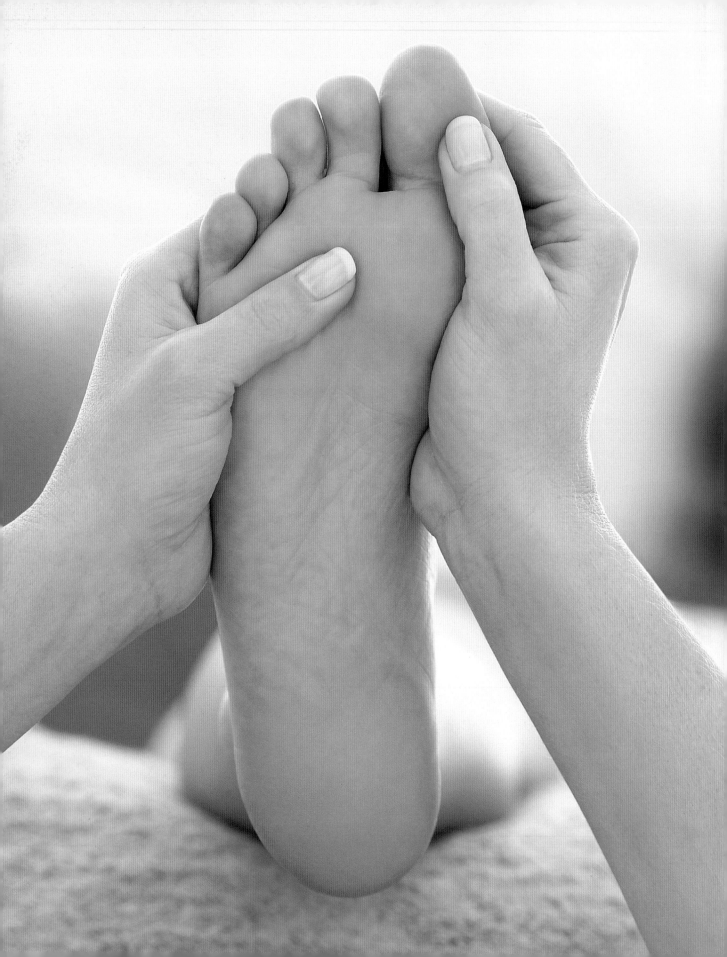

The basics of reflexology

Reflexology is a gentle and non-invasive way of healing, used to combat disease and encourage the body to heal itself. Whether you have a particular health problem or you are simply looking for a way to reduce tension and feel better, reflexology may be the answer. It strengthens the immune system, detoxifies the body and brings total relaxation – this is important as it is when the body is in a stressed, tense state that illnesses are more likely to occur.

Reflexology can be used not only to treat diseases and dysfunctions of the body but also to maintain good health. It is a wonderful way to ease stress and is the first step towards a healthier lifestyle. In particular, reflexology can be of great benefit in treating many of the conditions that affect a woman's health – and quality of life – such as endometriosis, period pains, ovarian cysts and fertility problems. With the help of this natural therapy, women of all ages can find relief from both physical ailments and the symptoms of stress.

How reflexology works

Reflexology began in Ancient Egypt in 2330 BC and was used in China in conjunction with acupuncture as long ago as the 4th century BC. Chinese physicians would insert acupuncture needles, then apply a deep pressure therapy to the feet in order to enhance the flow of energy (*chi*) in the body along pathways called meridians. The therapy was introduced to the West in the 1930s by an American physiotherapist named Eunice Ingham, who refined its use for the modern world.

The basic principles of reflexology are that the feet contain thousands of nerve endings and every organ, function and part of the body has its relative reflex point in the foot. By working on these reflex points reflexology stimulates, through the nerve pathways, the organ function or body part that is tense, congested or damaged from an accident, injury, or illness. Reflexology breaks down any tension, helps the system to eliminate toxins where necessary, reduces pain quite dramatically and encourages the body to heal itself. Reflexology is also an aid to relaxation and a great way to reduce emotional stresses and strains.

Restoring health

For centuries people have used herbs for healing, as well as therapies such as meditation, visualization and relaxation to rid the mind of stresses and tension. To be 'ill at ease' causes diseases of the body to manifest and the natural system for curing disease is based on a return to nature. This can be achieved by means of a regulated diet, breathing exercises and the use of various therapies, such as reflexology, to stimulate the body and raise the vitality of the patient to a proper standard of health. Restoration of health does not necessarily have to come from a doctor, pills or surgery, but rather from the patient's own efforts to take care of themselves. The aim of therapies such as reflexology is to discover and eliminate the cause of disease and to use the most natural and least invasive methods to treat the whole person.

Reflexologists view good health as more than just the absence of disease. It is a vital dynamic state, enabling a person to thrive in, or adapt to, a wide range of environments and stresses. The therapeutic approach is basically twofold: to help individuals heal themselves (alas, most people still come to a reflexologist when they are sick; too few when they are still healthy). Even for those who are very seriously ill, reflexology can be an ideal complementary therapy, used alongside conventional treatment to help relax the patient and boost the immune system.

Impact of stress

Unfortunately today's society encourages many disease-promoting habits. While we all know we should stop smoking, take more exercise and reduce our stress levels, such lifestyle changes can be all too difficult to make in the face of peer group and commercial pressures.

High stress levels are common. The demands placed on us every day can build up to a point where it can feel almost impossible to cope. Job pressures, family arguments, financial worries, deadlines – these are common examples of stressors.

The body does have some basic control mechanisms geared towards counteracting the everyday pressures of life. However, if stress is extreme, and continues for a long period of time, we become exhausted. This affects our immune system and we may find that we succumb to constant colds and coughs more easily or to conditions such as high blood pressure, constipation or diarrhoea, headaches, heavy periods and menstrual pain. However, the body wants to be well and has remarkable powers for combating disease. Reflexology treatment can assist in this and is of great benefit for women of all ages.

Benefits of reflexology
Reflexology treatment helps to promote a sense of ease and well-being and is a pleasure both to give and receive. It helps to expel toxins, release tensions and restore the body's natural state of balance.

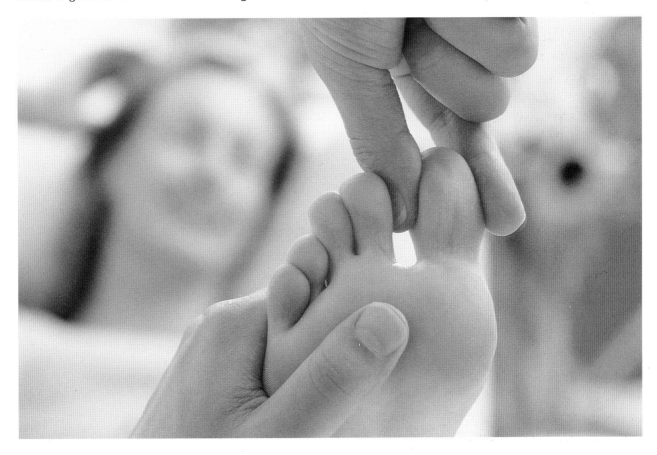

Solving problems with reflexology

If the body is suffering from inflammation, tension or congestion, the corresponding reflex points in the feet will reveal sensitivity when pressure is applied. In this way your feet can give an accurate picture of your health. The treatment is a deep pressure therapy, working on the tiny reflex points, mostly with the thumb, in a forwards creeping motion (see page 12). As these are stimulated, the flow of energy is restored and the body brought into balance once again. Relaxation techniques are also part of a treatment session (see pages 116–17).

Sensitivity in reflex points can warn of a weak spot in the body. If the imbalance is treated promptly with reflexology it can often be corrected and the illness avoided. Reflexology can also reveal past injuries, as any remaining scar tissue will cause sensitivity in the reflexes.

The feet really do reflect the human body, with the right foot governing the right side of the body and the left foot the left. The toes represent the head and sinus areas, eyes and ears. Below the toes are the reflex areas to the lungs, breasts and shoulders.

At the mid-line of the foot are links to the digestive system and the intestines, and to the urinary and reproductive systems. The reflexes in the feet flow in the same order as the parts of the body, with the top of

Hands and feet

There are reflexes on the hands and feet, but those on the hands are harder to isolate as the surface is smaller. The reflexes on the feet are also much more sensitive than those on the hands, making the treatment most effective.

Foot guidelines

The guidelines on the feet shown here help you identify which areas of the feet relate to which areas of the body. The lines simply divide the feet into broad sections. All reflex points are found within these guidelines. For example, the reflex points for the organs of elimination lie between the pelvic and waist lines. Below the pelvic line are the reflexes for the reproductive organs.

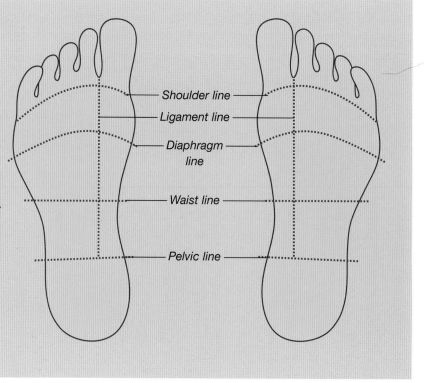

Shoulder line

Ligament line

Diaphragm line

Waist line

Pelvic line

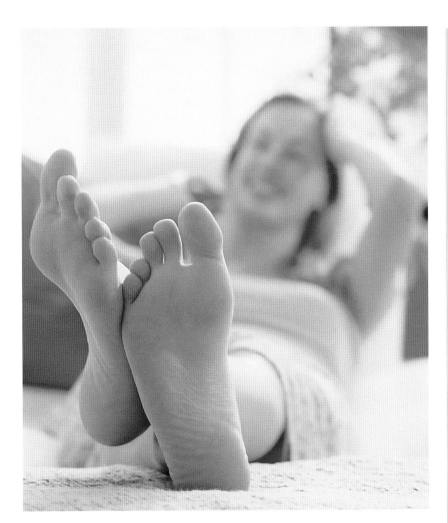

Views of the feet

The different areas of the feet are referred throughout this book as follows:

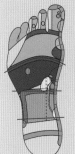

Plantar
This is the sole of the foot – the part you place down on the ground.

Dorsal
The top of the foot – the part you see when you look down at your feet.

Medial
The inside edge of the foot, in line with your big toe.

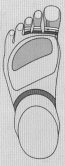

Lateral
The outside edge of the foot, in line with your little toe.

the feet relating to the upper part of the body and the lower parts of the feet to the organ functions and areas below the waist. The inside edge of the feet – the line from the inside of the heel right up to the inside of the big toe – relates to the vertebral column and central nervous system.

As the body begins to heal and symptoms are eased, the reflexes in the feet will become less sensitive. When sensitivity lessens or disappears altogether this is a sure sign that the body is healing and the person being treated is beginning to recover. She will notice a feeling of improved health and restored vitality. Most people also find that they sleep better after a treatment session.

It is safe to use reflexology in combination with other complementary therapies, such as aromatherapy, massage, acupuncture and shiatsu. And you can have reflexology while you are receiving homeopathic or herbal remedies, although you should always tell your practitioner what treatments you are having.

Reflexology techniques

Four basic techniques are used in reflexology. These are creeping, hooking out, rotating and spinal friction. Try to practise each one until you feel confident with the movement. The amount of pressure you use depends on the individual receiving the treatment – some people are happy with more pressure than others. Be sure to exert enough for the receiver to feel reaction in the reflex points, but not so much that it cases pain. A healthy person can generally cope with more pressure than someone who is elderly or unwell. For more advice on giving a complete foot treatment, see pages 114–23.

see pages 114–23.

Technique tips

• When giving reflexology, make sure your nails are clean and short. You should not be able to see them when you look at your hand palm up.

• Don't use massage oils when working the foot as it prevents proper contact with the reflexes and makes the skin too slippery. If the skin on the feet is very dry, smooth on a small amount of moisturizer.

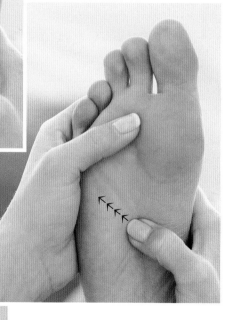

Creeping

The creeping movement is always forwards, never backwards. Move your thumb or finger across the foot in tiny methodical movements, rather like the way a caterpillar moves. Keep your thumb or finger flexed and work with the flat pad.

As you move your thumb, imagine that you are working across a pincushion full of pins. Each time you lift your thumb, creep it forwards a little and press as if you were pushing a pin into the pincushion.

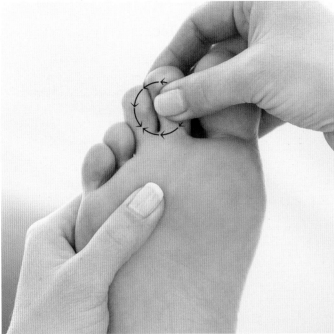

Rotating

This is used when certain reflex points need extra stimulation. Place the flat pad of your thumb on the reflex point and rotate it inwards, using small but firm movements. Keep the pressure up for several seconds for the greatest benefit.

Spinal friction

This is a special technique for stimulating and warming the spinal column. Place the palm of your hand on the medial (inside) edge of the foot, in line with the big toe. Rub your hand vigorously up and down.

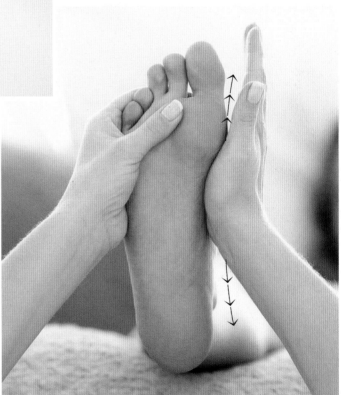

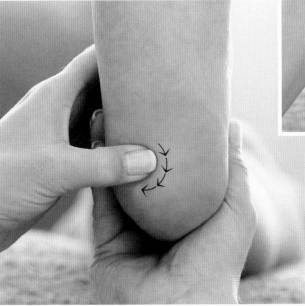

Hooking out

Use this technique to stimulate the ileocecal valve reflex. This valve joins the large and small intestines and the reflex point is on the lateral edge of the foot. Using your left thumb, press firmly on this point, then use the flat of your thumb to make an outwards-hooking movement in the shape of the letter 'j'.

Plantar foot map

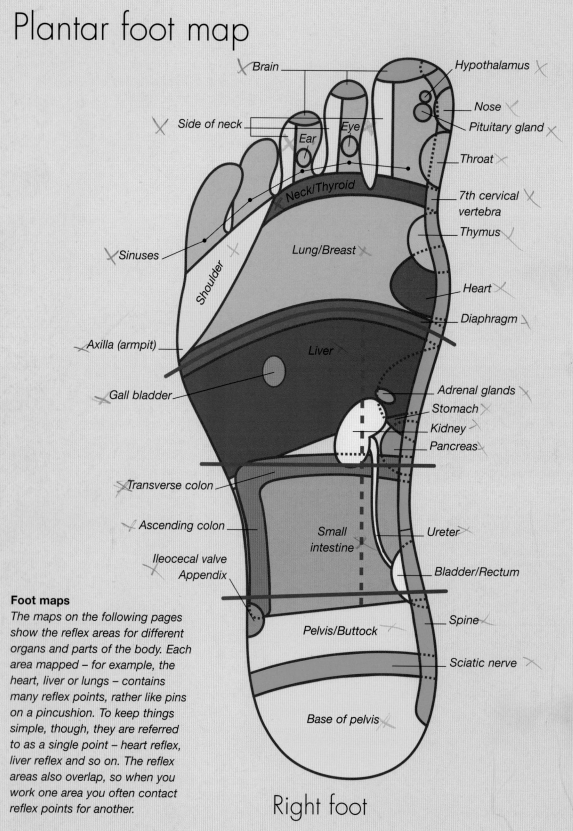

Brain

Hypothalamus

Nose

Side of neck

Eye

Pituitary gland

Ear

Throat

Neck/Thyroid

7th cervical vertebra

Thymus

Sinuses

Lung/Breast

Shoulder

Heart

Diaphragm

Axilla (armpit)

Liver

Gall bladder

Adrenal glands

Stomach

Kidney

Pancreas

Transverse colon

Ascending colon

Small intestine

Ureter

Ileocecal valve

Appendix

Bladder/Rectum

Spine

Pelvis/Buttock

Sciatic nerve

Base of pelvis

Right foot

Foot maps

The maps on the following pages
show the reflex areas for different
organs and parts of the body. Each
area mapped – for example, the
heart, liver or lungs – contains
many reflex points, rather like pins
on a pincushion. To keep things
simple, though, they are referred
to as a single point – heart reflex,
liver reflex and so on. The reflex
areas also overlap, so when you
work one area you often contact
reflex points for another.

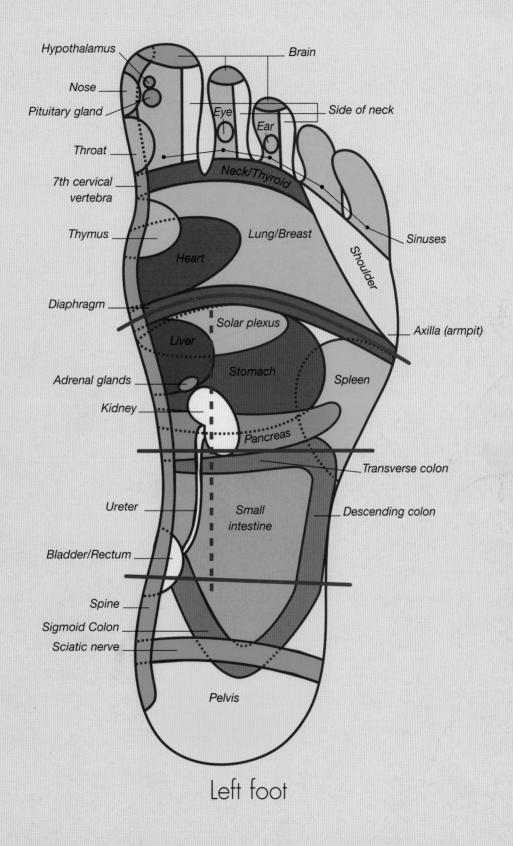

Hypothalamus

Brain

Nose

Pituitary gland

Eye

Side of neck

Ear

Throat

Neck/Thyroid

7th cervical
vertebra

Thymus

Lung/Breast

Sinuses

Heart

Shoulder

Diaphragm

Solar plexus

Liver

Axilla (armpit)

Stomach

Adrenal glands

Spleen

Kidney

Pancreas

Transverse colon

Ureter

Small
intestine

Descending colon

Bladder/Rectum

Spine

Sigmoid Colon

Sciatic nerve

Pelvis

Left foot

Dorsal foot map

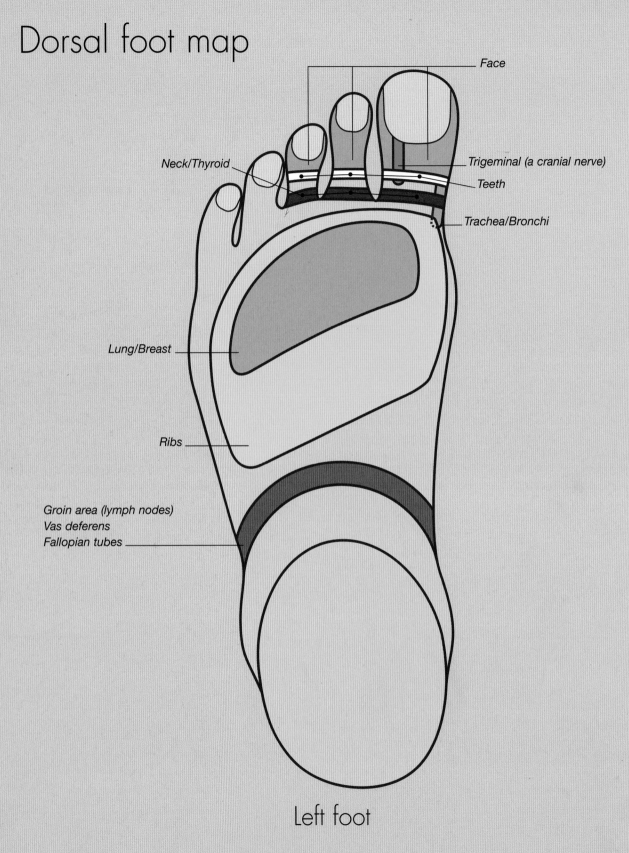

Face

Neck/Thyroid

Trigeminal (a cranial nerve)

Teeth

Trachea/Bronchi

Lung/Breast

Ribs

Groin area (lymph nodes)
Vas deferens
Fallopian tubes

Left foot

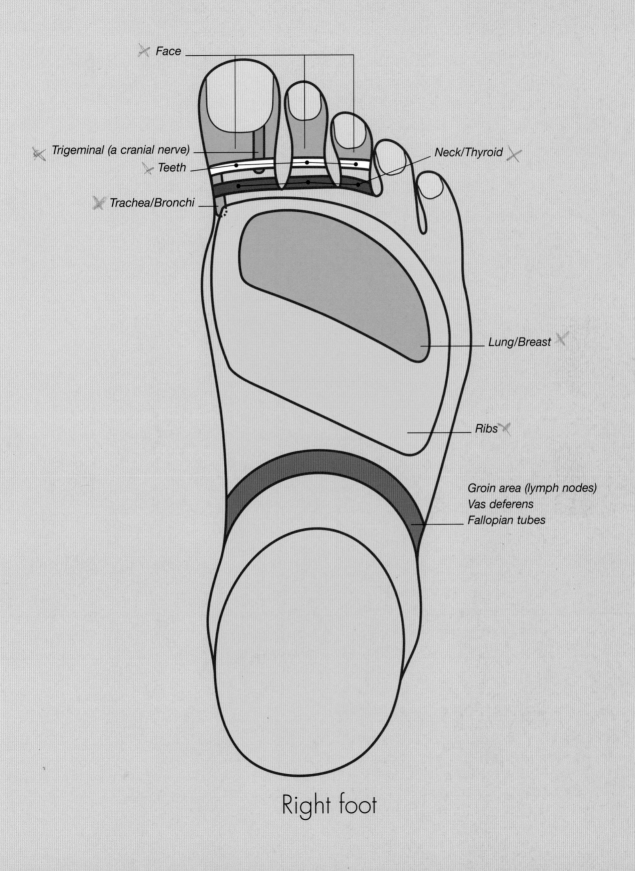

Face

Trigeminal (a cranial nerve)

Teeth

Trachea/Bronchi

Neck/Thyroid

Lung/Breast

Ribs

Groin area (lymph nodes)
Vas deferens
Fallopian tubes

Right foot

Medial and lateral foot maps

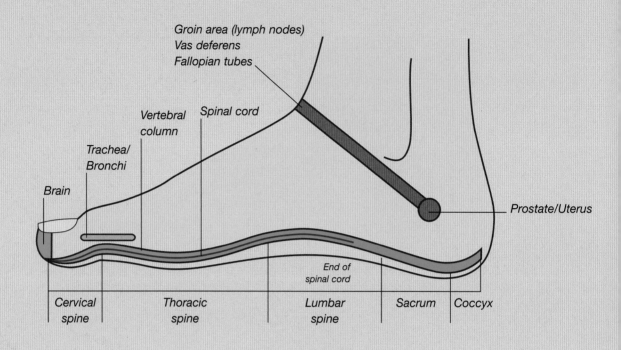

Groin area (lymph nodes)
Vas deferens
Fallopian tubes

Vertebral column

Spinal cord

Trachea/ Bronchi

Brain

Prostate/Uterus

End of spinal cord

| Cervical spine | Thoracic spine | Lumbar spine | Sacrum | Coccyx |

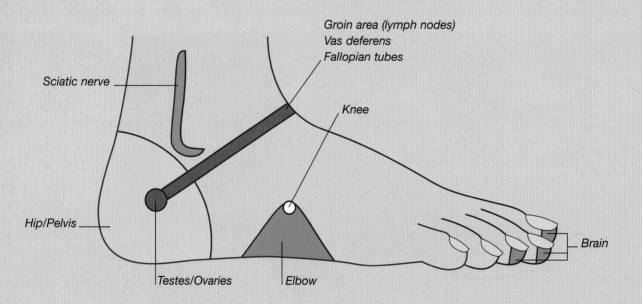

Groin area (lymph nodes)
Vas deferens
Fallopian tubes

Sciatic nerve

Knee

Hip/Pelvis

Brain

Testes/Ovaries

Elbow

Right foot

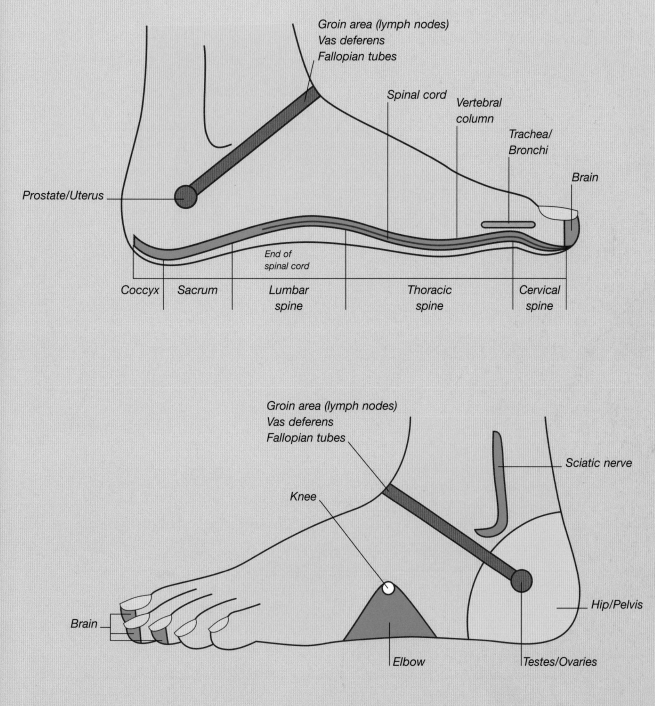

Groin area (lymph nodes)
Vas deferens
Fallopian tubes

Spinal cord

Vertebral
column

Trachea/
Bronchi

Brain

Prostate/Uterus

End of
spinal cord

Coccyx   Sacrum   Lumbar
spine

Thoracic
spine

Cervical
spine

Groin area (lymph nodes)
Vas deferens
Fallopian tubes

Sciatic nerve

Knee

Brain

Hip/Pelvis

Elbow

Testes/Ovaries

Left foot

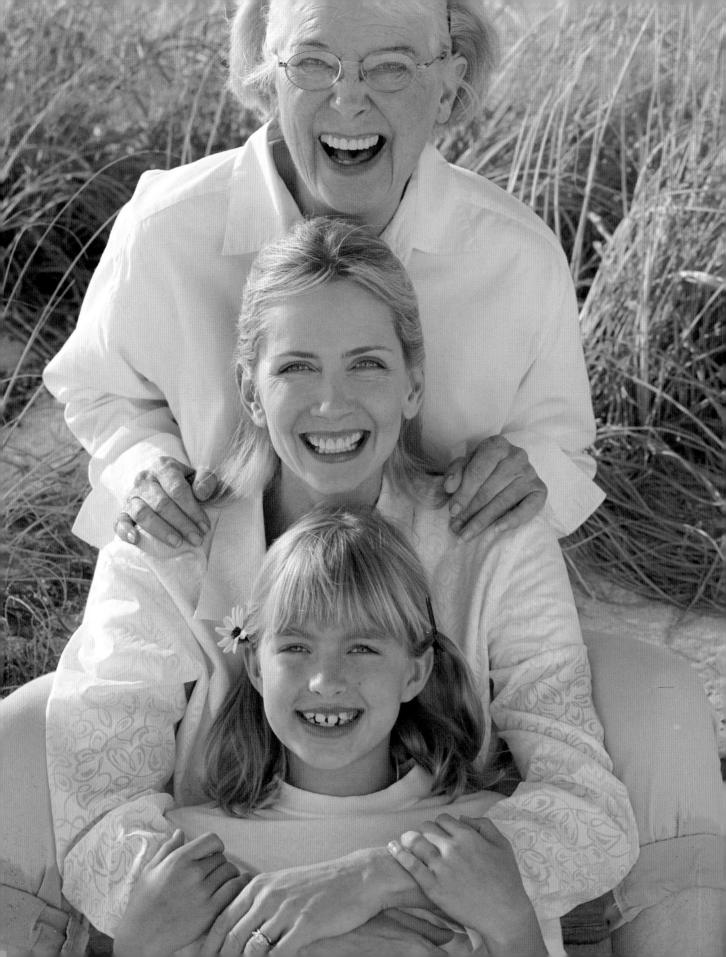

Reflexology for women of every age

Reflexology is the answer to many of the problems that affect a woman's health and lifestyle. Treatment can help everyone – from teenagers suffering from painful periods and women having trouble conceiving, to older women in the menopausal years, with symptoms such as hot flushes, mood swings and the depression and anxiety that accompany these hormonal changes. Reflexology can help with the emotional and physical discomforts of premenstrual tension, a condition that is all too common and affects three in ten women.

You may prefer to see a practitioner, particularly if you have a serious problem, but it is not difficult to follow the instructions in this book and swap treatment sessions with your friends or loved ones. To treat any of the conditions in this and the following chapters, follow the complete foot treatment on pages 114–23, then spend some extra time on the reflexes recommended for the condition. If time is short, you could try just working the reflexes for the particular ailment.

Always warm the foot up first, with the relaxation exercises on pages 116–17. Complete the whole sequence on the right foot before repeating the treatment on the left foot. As a preventative treatment, it is a good idea to have reflexology at least once a month.

Menstrual problems

Reflexology can bring relief from the discomforts of premenstrual tension and help to treat conditions such as heavy periods and endometriosis.

Menorrhagia (heavy periods)

Problems with excessive menstrual bleeding or menorrhagia can be eased by dietary measures, combined with regular sessions of reflexology. As with any disease, proper determination of the cause is essential for effective treatment.

One cause of menorrhagia may involve abnormalities in the biochemical processes of the endometrium (the lining of the uterus), which controls the supply of arachidonic acid, a fatty acid from which prostaglandins are derived. This type of prostaglandin can lead to increased blood flow and a reduced blood-clotting ability. Research shows that women suffering from menorrhagia have higher than normal levels of arachidonic acid. It is thought that this excess of prostaglandin activity is the cause of both menstrual cramps and excessive bleeding.

Factors that may contribute to this condition are low thyroid activity, vitamin A deficiency, and intrauterine devices. Other causes include endometrial polyps and endometriosis, so always check with your doctor so that any of these problems can be ruled out.

Keep moving

Regular exercise such as swimming and brisk walking may help to reduce symptoms of menorrhagia and other menstrual problems.

Self-help

Some simple changes to your diet and the addition of certain supplements can help reduce menorrhagia.

• Make sure your diet is relatively low in sources of arachidonic acid (animal fats) and high in linolenic acid (vegetable oils). Eat green leafy vegetables, such as spinach, cabbage and brussels sprouts.

• Iron supplements are a preventative therapy and women during their menstruating/child-bearing years should take a daily iron supplement to avoid deficiency.

• In one study, vitamin A levels were found to be significantly lower in women with menorrhagia. After taking prescribed doses of vitamin A twice daily for 15 days blood loss returned to normal.

• Herbal treatments of menorrhagia include blue cohosh, witch hazel and shepherd's purse. Shepherd's purse has a long history of general use in obstetrics and is of significant help.

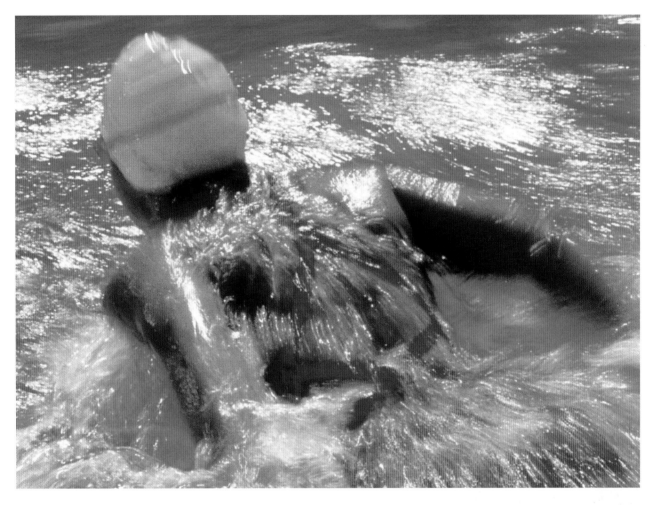

Endometriosis

In this condition, endometrial cells, which normally grow in the uterus, escape and grow abnormally in the pelvic cavity. The endometrial cells cluster together and attach themselves to any part of the pelvic cavity, ovaries, fallopian tubes, bladder or bowel, and sometimes other parts of the body, causing excessive congestion and bleeding. The woman's fertility is usually affected because the endometrial tissue on the ovary can block the release of eggs and strangle the delicate tubes that carry the egg to the womb.

Endometriosis is a major cause of menstrual pain and is becoming increasingly common. It also affects fertility. It is estimated that 40–60 per cent of women who undergo hysterectomies have endometriosis, even if this is not the main reason for surgery. The endometrial cells outside the uterus respond to the normal menstrual cycle. Thus the tissue may actually lessen by the time the woman is examined only to proliferate again as her oestrogen levels change during her menstrual cycle.

Self-help

If you are suffering from endometriosis, take a daily B-complex vitamin supplement (20 to 75 milligrams) in addition to 1000 milligrams of choline and 500 milligrams of inositol. These two nutrients are part of the B-complex but seem to be most important in liver function.

Regular aerobic exercise such as jogging, swimming or cycling, or a work-out in the gym stimulates the release of endorphins. These are natural opiates that produce a sense of well-being and block pain perception.

B-complex to the rescue

There are a number of theories as to the cause of endometriosis, including hormonal imbalances, stress and deficiencies in certain nutrients. B vitamins are particularly important as they help to reduce the intensity of menstrual pain and re-balance hormones. They also support the liver, which processes oestrogen. B-complex vitamins are found in meats, fish, eggs, dairy products, pulses and brewer's yeast. Wholegrains are also a source of Vitamin B. Citrus fruits, which are rich in bioflavonoids, can cause endometrial flare-ups if eaten in excess.

Stress rapidly depletes the body of B vitamins, as does having too much refined carbohydrate and alcohol, which rob tissues of nutrients in the process of being metabolized. White sugar is the worst culprit.

Polycystic ovary syndrome (PCOS)

The cysts on polycystic ovaries are in fact clumps of undeveloped follicles. They do not always cause problems, but there can be symptoms such as infrequent or absent periods, excess hair on the face and body, acne, weight problems and mood swings. Blood tests will reveal a hormone imbalance. One cause of PCOS may be a high level of blood insulin, which disrupts normal ovulation.

There are all manner of surgical interventions and drug therapies available, but these are not without side-effects and do not deal with the cause of the condition. The first step for a PCOS sufferer is to lose weight if necessary. As weight is reduced hormone levels start to return to normal and ovarian function is improved.

Ovarian cysts

Many women develop growths known as cysts in or on their ovaries. Most of these cysts are filled with a watery fluid and may erupt of their own accord, causing no problems. You are more likely to develop ovarian cysts if you are between 20 and 35, have not had children, smoke, and drink more

Self-help

If you are suffering from polycystic ovary syndrome, there are some dietary changes and supplements that may help.

• Eat foods containing natural oestrogen, such as chickpeas and soya products.

• Eat regular meals so that your body does not have dramatic changes in blood sugar levels. Surges in blood sugar levels affect your hormonal functions.

• Be aware that all stimulating foods and drinks such as tea, coffee, cola drinks, alcohol and chocolate stimulate the adrenal glands. When over-stimulated, the adrenal glands will produce an excess of androgens, which are male hormones, and an excess of this hormone can affect ovulation.

• Take chromium, an important supplement for PCOS sufferers as it helps control blood sugar levels and regulates insulin in the body.

Eat to balance your hormones

Many hormonal imbalances are caused or made worse by an excess of oestrogen in the body, so it is a good idea to watch what you eat very carefully and adopt a hormone-balancing diet. The following dietary tips will help balance your hormones and ease most hormone-related conditions.

EAT FRESH ORGANIC FOOD
Eat plenty of fresh fruit and vegetables – at least five servings a day and more if you can manage. Also eat wholegrains, such as oats, wholemeal bread and brown rice. Choose organic foods where possible.

EAT OILY FISH, NUTS AND SEEDS
Include oily fish, such as herrings, mackerel and sardines, in your diet as well as nuts and seeds – sunflower seeds and pumpkin seeds are delicious sprinkled on a bowl of cereal or salad. Use olive oil as a salad dressing or in your cooking.

WATER
Drink plenty of water and diluted fruit juices.

FIBRE
Increase the amount of fibre in your diet. If you are prone to constipation, take physillium husks mixed with water twice daily. These husks swell up in the bowel and encourage toxins to be absorbed from the walls of the bowel and eliminated with ease.

CHECK TINNED AND PACKAGED FOODS
Get used to reading labels on tinned and packaged foods before you buy them and avoid additives, preservatives and artificial sweeteners.

REDUCE CAFFEINE
Try not to have too much caffeine. Remember that caffeine is not only in tea and coffee, it is also in chocolate and chocolate-based products as well as in cola drinks.

AVOID SUGAR
Avoid sugar, whether brown or white. It is of no value to the body whatsoever, and causes huge surges of insulin into our bloodstream.

TAKE VITAMIN AND MINERALS
• Take garlic, preferably as a daily supplement. It has a positive effect on cells.
• Zinc plays an important role in the reproductive system. It is necessary for normal egg development and for the production of healthy sperm in the male.
• B Vitamins are needed by your liver, which is a great detoxifier, to rid the body of excessive amounts of oestrogen.
• False unicorn root has been shown to improve the functioning of the ovaries.
• Echinacea boosts the immune system and can also help the body to destroy abnormal cells.

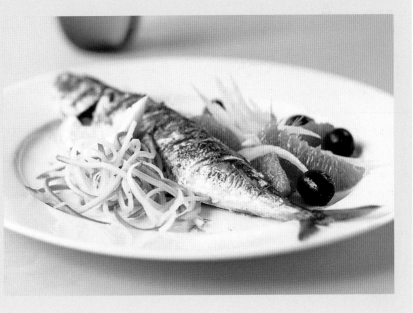

Oily fish
Even one meal of oily fish a week has clear health benefits, which outweigh the risks from any pollution in the fish. Current advice is to eat oily fish up to four times a week. However, pregnant and breastfeeding women should eat only two portions a week.

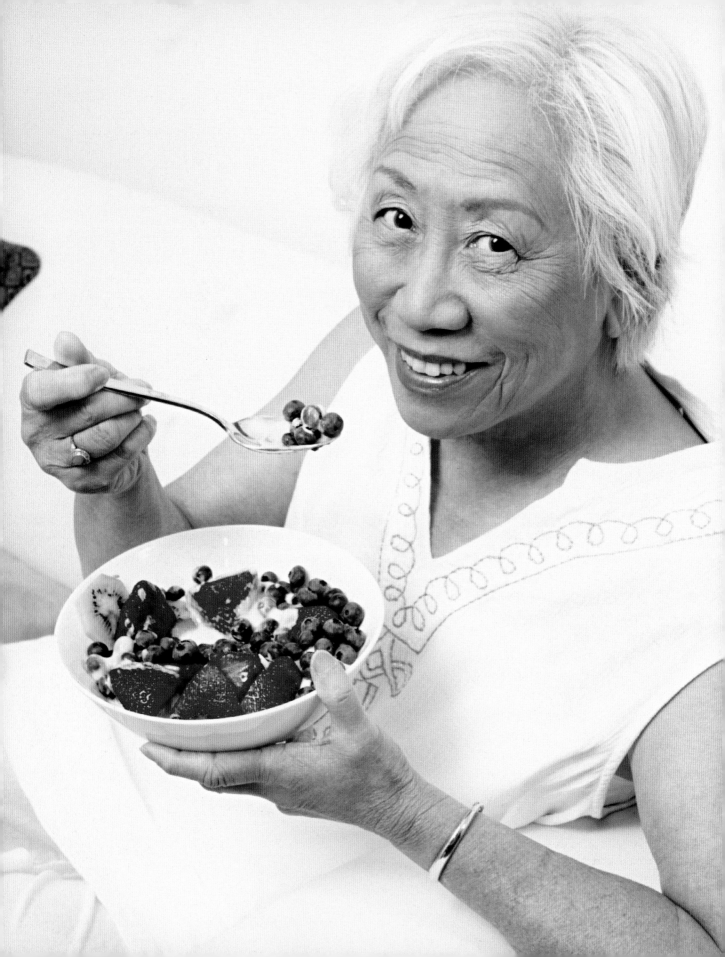

than three units of alcohol a day. Some women have ovarian cysts and are totally unaware of them. Others experience irregular periods, pain, a dull ache in the side, pain during intercourse, breakthrough bleeding and enlargement of the abdomen.

Cysts can grow extremely large and cause pressure and pain in the pelvic cavity, affecting the menstrual cycle. It is important to have a diagnosis if a cyst is discovered, as there is just a chance it could be cancerous. Some types of cyst disappear of their own accord; some need treatment. In any case, you need to re-balance your hormones with the help of nutrition and supplements. See the dietary advice on page 25 and see pages 28–29 for the reflexology treatments that can help balance your hormones and boost liver health.

Premenstrual tension

For most women PMT starts after the middle of the cycle (ovulation) and ceases just as soon as the period arrives. Symptoms are varied, but may include irritability, anxiety, breast tenderness, water retention, weight gain, headaches, food cravings and tiredness. More women suffer accidents both in the home and on the road in this premenstrual phase than at any other time.

-- No real conclusions have been reached, despite extensive research, as to what causes these symptoms. We know that there is an excess of oestrogen circulating in the bloodstream at this time that would account for the fluid retention, irritability and breast pain. PMT is more common in women in the 25–35 age range and in those who have had children. It is also more common after miscarriage or coming off the contraceptive pill.

Keep active and eat well
Having a good diet and plenty of exercise is excellent advice for everyone, but particularly beneficial for women suffering from any kind of menstrual complaint.

Self-help

If you suffer from distressing PMT symptoms every month, try these tips.

• Take evening primrose oil supplement regularly. Some women find it very helpful for easing symptoms, particularly breast pain.

• Cut down on salt, sugar, caffeine and alcohol and eat more fibre and fresh foods (see page 25).

• Keep your blood sugar steady by eating little and often.

• Take regular exercise, even when you have PMT – you will find it helps.

Cervical cancer

This serious condition seems to be on the increase. There are many theories on the reasons for this, but it seems increasingly likely that cervical cancer is mainly due to viral infection. Research also shows that smoking doubles your chances of developing abnormal cervical cell changes. It is interesting to note that folic acid deficiency can cause abnormal changes in the cells of the cervix.

This cancer can be treated very successfully, but the earlier it is diagnosed the better. There may be no symptoms, but cervical smear tests pick up any cell changes at a very early stage so it is essential to have these regularly. If there are any signs of abnormal cells you will need to have a follow-up test six months later, but very often these cells will have returned to normal. It is a good idea for women with a history of abnormal cells to take folic acid tablets on a regular and permanent basis.

All women should start having cervical smears once they begin having sexual intercourse and continue to be tested every three years up to the age of 65.

Anyone with cervical cancer will, of course, be treated by a medical practitioner, but reflexology can be a useful supporting treatment of benefit to the whole body.

General treatments

The reflexology treatments shown on these pages and pages 30–31 can all help ease menorrhagia, endometriosis, polycystic ovary syndrome, ovarian cysts and premenstrual tension. They can also be used as complementary therapy for more serious conditions, such as cervical cancer, in addition to orthodox medical treatment. Work on the reflexes relating to the reproductive organs will bring relief, but you also need to pay attention to the endocrine system by working on the pituitary and thyroid reflexes to correct hormonal imbalances. The liver is the body's great detoxifier, so work on the liver reflex helps rid the body of toxins that can cause hormone imbalances.

Areas to work

- Liver
- Pituitary
- Thyroid
- Ovaries
- Fallopian tubes
- Uterus
- Breast – for premenstrual tension

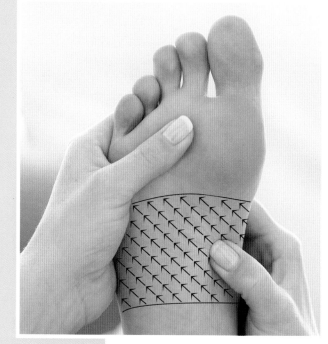

Try these supplements

These supplements may help reduce your PMT symptoms.

• Take a daily calcium and magnesium supplement. Magnesium has a calming effect on the nervous system.

• Take a zinc supplement. Zinc plays an important part in the action of our hormonal system and many women with premenstrual syndrome have low levels of zinc in their bloodstream.

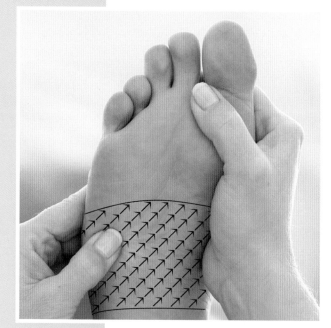

Liver
The liver reflex is only on the right foot. Holding the foot with your left hand, creep across the reflex area with your right thumb. Work from the medial to the lateral side at the angle shown (top). Switch hands and work back across the area in the opposite direction (above).

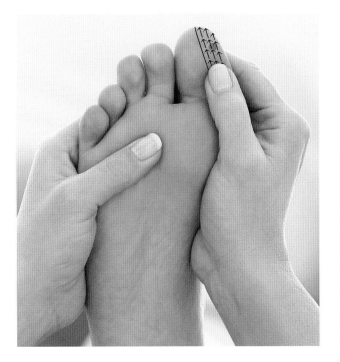

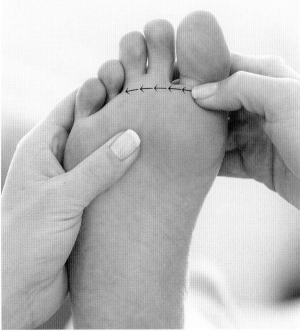

Pituitary

Hold the right foot with your left hand. Starting at the base, creep up the big toe with your right thumb. Change hands to work the left foot.

Thyroid (plantar)

Hold the right foot with your left hand. Use your right thumb to creep along the bases of the first three toes.

Thyroid (dorsal)

Hold the right foot with your left fist. With your right index finger, creep along the base of the first three toes. Repeat three times. Change hands to treat the left foot.

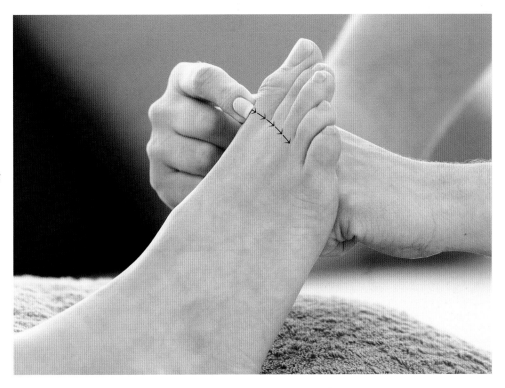

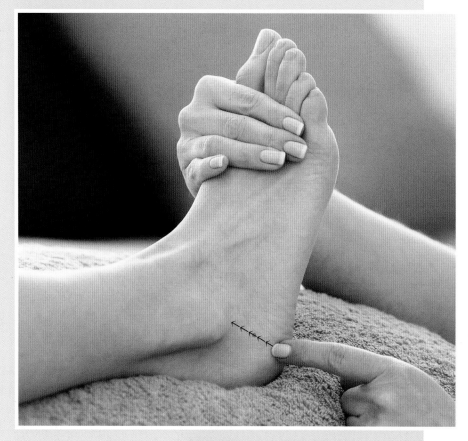

Ovaries

Hold the right foot with your right hand. The reflex point for the ovaries is between the heel and the ankle bone on the lateral side of the foot, so use your left index finger to creep from the tip of the heel to the ankle bone. Change hands to work the left foot.

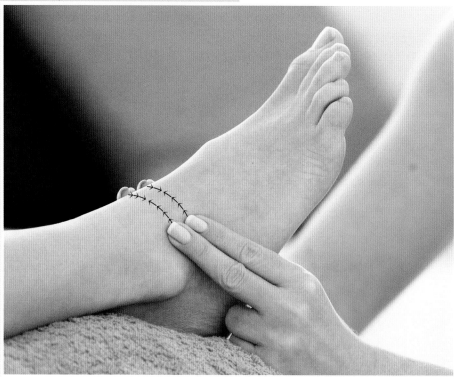

Fallopian tubes

Using both your thumbs, press into the sole of the right foot. At the same time, creep across the top of the foot with the index and third fingers of both hands. Repeat this two or three times. Work the left foot in the same way.

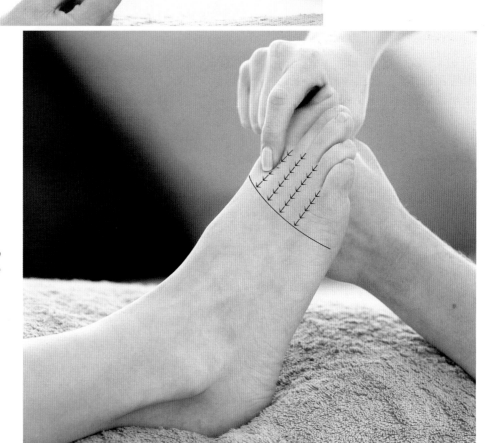

Uterus

Hold the right foot with your left hand. The reflex point for the uterus is between the heel and the ankle bone on the medial side, so work across this area from the tip of the heel with your right index finger. Change hands to work the left foot.

Breast

Push your left fist into the sole of the right foot. Using your right index finger, creep down the grooves below the toes on the top of the foot. Change hands to work the left foot.

Treating candida

The common yeast *Candida albicans* is present in everyone. Normally the yeast lives harmlessly in certain parts of the body, including the mouth and the vagina, but occasionally it overgrows and causes problems. The areas that are most sensitive to the yeast are the gastro-intestinal and genito-urinary systems. Some allergies are also attributed to candida overgrowth.

Candida can be a side-effect of antibiotic use, when good bacteria as well as bad are destroyed. Antibiotics can be life-saving, but in my view they are used too freely today for quite minor conditions, which would resolve themselves within a few days with simple home remedies and rest. We also take in antibiotics, unknowingly, through food, as they are used to prevent disease in meat and poultry.

Candida in the intestinal tract can also be the result of other drugs, such as corticosteroids, anti-ulcer drugs, oral contraceptive pills, lack of digestive secretions or too much sugar in the diet.

Areas to work

- Stomach
- Liver
- Intestines

Self-help

• Pay strict attention to what you eat and drink. Avoid all forms of sugar, including fruit juices and honey. Avoid milk and milk products too, due to their high content of lactose (milk sugar) and trace levels of antibiotics.

• Eliminate all known allergens since allergies can weaken the immune system and provide the ideal environment for the yeast to thrive.

• Take lactobacillus in capsule form to help restore a healthy balance in the intestinal area.

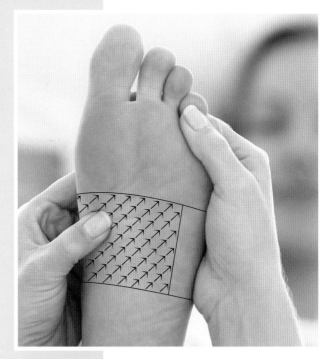

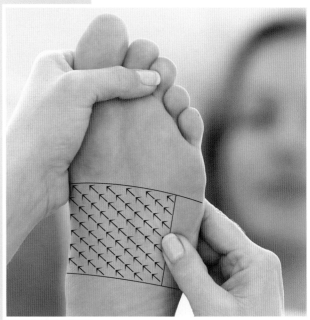

Stomach
This reflex is only on the left foot. Supporting the left foot with your right hand, work over the area with your left thumb from the medial to the lateral side of the foot (top). Switch hands and work back again with your right thumb (above).

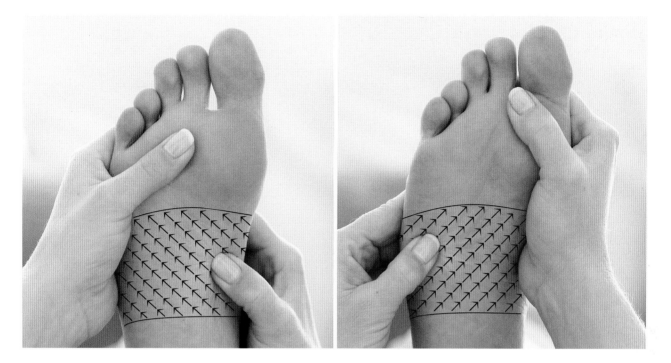

Liver

The liver reflex is only on the right foot. Holding the foot with your left hand, creep across the reflex area with your right thumb. Work from the medial to the lateral side at the angle shown (above left). Switch hands and work back across the area in the opposite direction (above right).

Intestines

Support the right foot with your left hand. Using your right thumb, work over the area below the waist line (see p. 10) with your right thumb, moving in straight lines from the medial to the lateral side (right). Change hands and use your left thumb to work back from the lateral to the medial side (far right). Then, work the left foot starting with your left thumb.

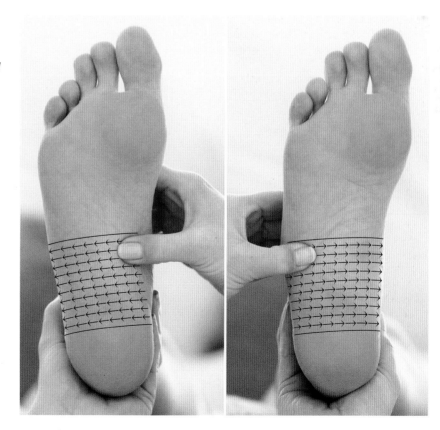

Treating cystitis

Bladder infections in women are very common and about 21 per cent of all women have urinary tract discomfort at least once a year. The painful and disabling symptoms can become chronic. The inflammation in the lining of the bladder causes burning pain on urination, frequent need to urinate, and excessive need to urinate at night. Foul-smelling or dark urine and lower abdominal pain are further unpleasant symptoms. Many factors are associated with an increased risk of bladder infections, including pregnancy, sexual intercourse, mechanical trauma or irritation. Some women also have structural abnormalities of the urinary tract that block the free flow of urine.

Area to work
• Urinary system

Self-help

• Wearing tight-fitting jeans and synthetic underwear makes cystitis worse. Wear cotton underwear always and loose clothing when suffering from an infection. Years ago, when women wore wool or cotton underwear and skirts that allowed air to circulate more freely, cystitis was almost unknown.

• Drink plenty of water – at least three litres a day – and avoid alcohol, strong tea and coffee while suffering from cystitis.

• Drink cranberry juice, too – two or three glasses a day at the first sign of symptoms. It reduces the ability of the bacteria to adhere or stick to the lining of the bladder and urethra.

• Garlic is known to have an anti-microbial action against many disease-causing organisms, cystitis being one.

• Take vitamin C, up to 500 mg three times a day, and vitamin A.

• Urinate after intercourse. Women who have a tendency to suffer from bladder infections should wash their labia and urethra before and after intercourse to eliminate all possible bacterial invasion from their partner.

• Hold a hot-water bottle over your lower abdomen. The warmth can be very comforting.

• Don't use perfumed bubble bath liquid and soaps. They can cause irritation.

Why not try?

Goldenseal – it is one of the most effective of the herbal anti-microbial agents. It has a long history of use by naturopathic physicians and herbalists for the treatment of infections and is well documented in scientific literature.

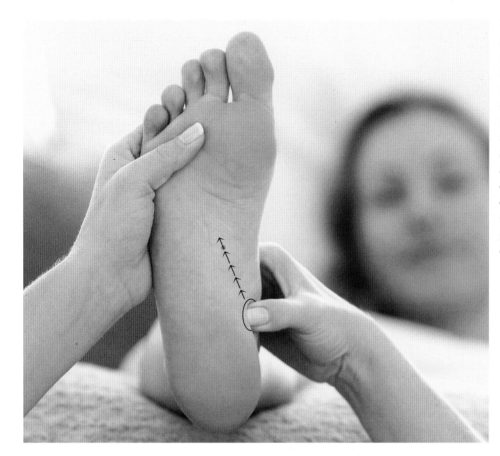

Urinary system

Support the top of the right foot with your left hand. Using your right thumb, creep up the inside edge of the ligament line to the waist line (see page 10). Don't work on the ligament itself. Contact the kidney reflex, which lies just above where the waist and ligament lines intersect (see page 10), and rotate with your thumb. Change hands to treat the left foot.

System-boosting hand treatment

This gives a general boost to the whole system and is a treatment you can give yourself. Support your hand on a small cushion or a pillow. Use the thumb of your other hand to creep up the whole spinal reflex from the base of the hand up to the top of the thumb. Change hands and repeat the treatment.

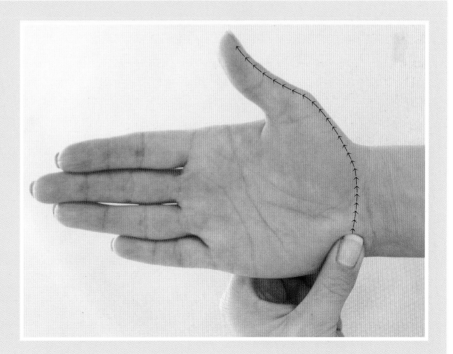

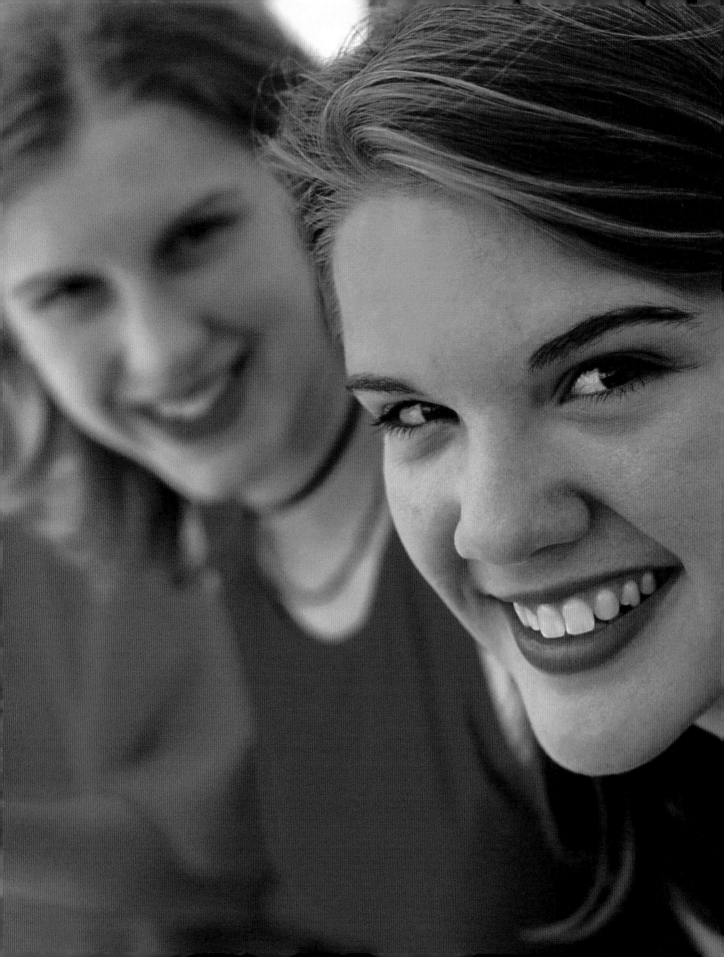

Reflexology during the teenage years

Being a teenager can be a bewildering time as you struggle with a range of physical and emotional changes, as well as emerging sexuality and personal insecurities. Most teenage girls experience swings of emotion that can be hard to cope with – for other family members and for teenagers themselves.

Changing from being a little girl, dependent on your family, into an adult with so many demands being made upon you, is not easy. During these years there are many stresses – examinations to study for, worries about relationships, insecurity about personal appearance, and often peer pressure to smoke, drink or take drugs.

During all this emotional upheaval, reflexology can be invaluable. An angry, confused teenager can respond surprisingly well to this healing hands-on treatment offered by a parent, friend or practitioner. One of the major benefits of treatment is probably to reduce high levels of stress, which can in turn exacerbate other conditions such as acne, painful periods and headaches. Reflexology can also help balance the hormonal system, which is of prime importance during the teenage years when dramatic changes in the body's hormonal balance are taking place.

Teenage problems

Hormones are at the root of most teenage health problems. Here are some of the most common, all of which can be helped by reflexology.

Acne

At a time when appearance is all-important, this is a particularly distressing condition. Pus-filled spots, blackheads and reddish lumps appear on the face, chest and back, caused by an excess of oil in the sebaceous glands, which seems to block the pores.

The sebaceous glands in the skin produce an oily substance called sebum, which lubricates the skin and prevents excessive water loss. If too much sebum is generated the pores can become blocked and the skin inflamed and infected. The activity of the sebaceous glands is controlled by male sex hormones called androgens. Acne often first appears during puberty when there is an increase in the production of sex hormones in both girls and boys.

Some doctors prescribe long-term antibiotics for acne. These relieve, but do not cure, the problem. They can cause damage to the intestinal area as they destroy the flora of the bowel, which keeps the balance between the bacterial levels. Long-term antibiotic use also affects the immune system. Many naturopaths believe that poor elimination is at the root of skin problems, so it really is important to make sure that you open

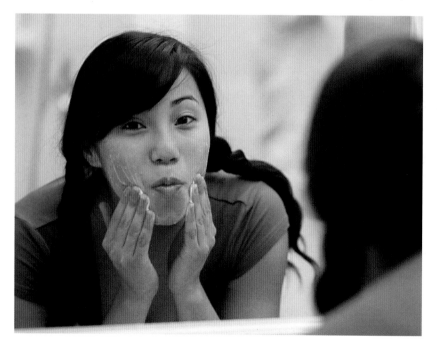

Keep clean
To keep your skin looking good, cleanse your face thoroughly morning and night, whether you have spots or not. Drinking plenty of water helps keep your skin healthy too.

Self-help

Research indicates that what you eat does not cause or cure acne, but a good diet will certainly improve general health and well-being and assist recovery. Supplements have also been shown to be of some benefit for sufferers.

EAT WELL
A good diet, low in fat and high in fibre, helps. Eat lots of vegetables and fruits – raw whenever possible – and drink plenty of pure mineral water and herbal or fruit teas. Certain types of dietary fibre are particularly good at absorbing toxins and eliminating them from the bowel, so include some wholegrains, pulses and jacket potatoes in your diet.

FATTY ACIDS
Fresh seeds, nuts and cold-pressed vegetable oils are rich in essential fatty acids, so eat these instead of saturated and hydrogenated fats.

SUGAR
Sugar has an immune-suppressing effect (and therefore inhibits resistance to bacterial infection), so all concentrated sugars should be eliminated from the diet. It is best to restrict all other refined carbohydrates (white flour, white rice, biscuits and cakes), too, as far as you can as well as fried foods and animal fats.

VITAMIN A
Vitamin A is one of the most important vitamins for skin health and has frequently been shown in studies to reduce the over-production of both sebum and keratin. Large doses are potentially toxic, however, so should only be taken under supervision.

ZINC
Zinc is a valuable supplement for acne sufferers as it is involved in the activation of hormones, wound healing, effective functioning of the immune system, control of inflammation and tissue regeneration.

HERBS
Echinacea inhibits inflammation, promotes wound healing, stimulates the immune system and kills bacteria. Goldenseal is also an effective herbal treatment for acne and other skin conditions.

Milk thistle aids the liver's detoxification process and helps protect the liver from damage. It is therefore a valuable addition to any treatment programme for skin conditions. It is when the liver does not cope adequately with detoxification that greater numbers of toxins are eliminated via the skin.

Garlic is a natural antiseptic, so take a daily supplement to reduce any inflammation on the skin. Steam facials infused with herbs give the skin a deep cleanse and encourages good skin care.

your bowels regularly. Any toxins retained in the bowel have to find their way out through other parts of the body.

Reflexology is of great benefit in helping the detoxification of the bowel and liver, so these two areas are vital to work on in order to get an all-round improvement in this upsetting condition.

Painful periods

It's quite common for periods to be painful at first until a regular menstrual cycle has been established. Much of the pain may be due to high levels of bad prostaglandins. These hormone-like chemicals can cause inflammation and pain and are often stimulated in the teenage years. Fortunately, there are also good prostaglandins that counteract inflammation and relax the muscles. An increased intake of linoleic acid (an essential fatty acid), which is found in sunflower and sesame seeds, walnuts, linseed and soya, helps boost levels of good prostaglandins and lessen period pain. Regular reflexology also helps relax the painful muscle spasms in the uterus.

Stress headaches

Many young people spend hours working at computers. Whether engaged in school or college or playing computer games, there is a great deal of strain and pressure on the neck and upper spine that causes pain in the shoulders, arms, neck and head.

If you spend long periods at a computer, check that your back is well supported and the computer screen in a good position so that you do not have to raise your head to look at the screen. Make sure that your hands and wrists are well supported – wrist supports take the pressure off your hands when you need to work for hours on a keyboard.

Teenage worries

Young girls face a lot of pressure today to look good, to be as skinny as the latest supermodel. Magazines have endless features about weight-loss diets – one minute they say low-fat, high-carbohydrate is best; next, high-protein and low-carbohydrate is all the rage.

Teenagers, and even children as young as eight or nine years old, are watching their figures, responding to the perceived message that in order to be beautiful you need to be thin. The increase in these pressures has resulted in eating disorders such as anorexia nervosa and bulimia.

Young women with anorexia see a fat woman when they look in the mirror, although they are really painfully thin. They have an obsessional fear of weight gain which takes control of their life and they may actually reduce their food intake to the point of near starvation. Some also exercise to excess, as they need to make absolutely sure that any food they eat will be 'burnt off' by exercise.

Women with bulimia also believe that they are overweight, but they overeat at times to such a degree that they lose control of what goes into their mouths. They eat anything and everything, even foods they intensely dislike. Following a period of overeating they self-induce vomiting and use large quantities of laxatives in an attempt to rid their body of the excess of foods. There is usually an associated reaction of self-loathing as they indulge in these periods of overeating.

Research has found that many of the sufferers of anorexia and bulimia are deficient in zinc. When zinc supplementation is given the eating disorders significantly improve.

Anorexia and bulimia are serious medical conditions and need very careful treatment by a specialist in the field. Reflexology is of great benefit in helping to reduce stress levels in these individuals, but I must stress that medical help from doctors experienced in the management of these disorders must always be sought.

Drinking and smoking

Being a non-smoker and keeping alcohol intake low will go a long way to keeping you healthy. Alcohol takes its toll on your liver and can compromise its ability to detoxify your system – one of the liver's main roles. One or two glasses of wine or beer are fine, on occasion, but heavy drinking sessions while you are still growing play havoc with your liver.

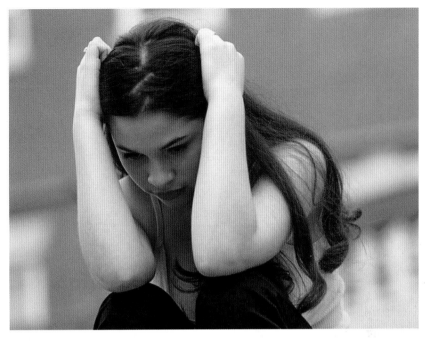

Calming your nerves
Nerve-wracking events such as examinations can be hard to face. A reflexology treatment the night before something such as an exam or an interview can calm and relax you, so you have a good night's sleep and you are ready to do your best.

Alcohol also affects your blood sugar levels and acts as an anti-nutrient, which means that it blocks the good effects of your food by depleting vitamins and minerals. It can also interfere with the metabolism of fatty acids which are absolutely crucial for good health. Apart from having a high toxic level when taken in excess, alcohol is also full of calories – a glass of wine contains about 100 calories and a pint of beer is around 200. If you are trying to watch your weight, remember that alcohol in excess can pile on the pounds.

Smoking, too, is disastrous for your health and well-being. Apart from making you smell unpleasant, it ages your skin faster than anything else. And you are 86 per cent more likely to develop cancer if you smoke. Cancer in the throat, mouth and lungs are far more common in smokers than non-smokers, as are cancer of the cervix, ovaries and bladder. Smoking also places an enormous strain on your heart and so your body is starved of essential oxygen-rich blood, which should reach every cell and keep you fit.

Regular reflexology treatment can help you maintain a respect for your body and resist temptations. You may prefer to see someone outside the family, but exchanging reflexology with your parents can be a safe, acceptable way of making caring contact.

Treating acne

Acne is particularly common in teenagers because of greatly increased levels of hormones which affect the amount of an oily substance called sebum in the skin. This can block sebaceous glands, causing blackheads and inflammation. Many women also suffer acne before their periods.

Reflexology is of great benefit in helping the detoxification of the bowel and liver, so these two areas are vital to work on in order to get an all-round improvement in this distressing skin condition.

Areas to work

- Liver
- Intestines
- Stomach

Self-help

- *Keep skin very clean, using a gentle cleansing product or an antiseptic soap.*

- *Always wash your hands before touching your face to prevent the spread of bacteria.*

- *Never squeeze pimples – it only makes them worse. You can very gently squeeze out blackheads after steaming your face to open pores.*

- *It's fine to wear make-up to cover your spots if it makes you feel better. It won't make the spots any worse, as long as you clean the make-up off carefully every evening.*

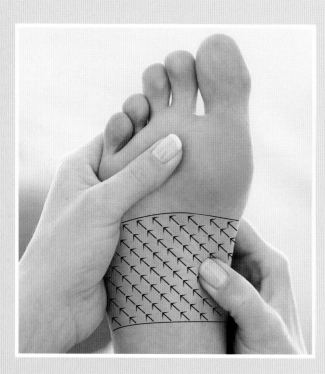

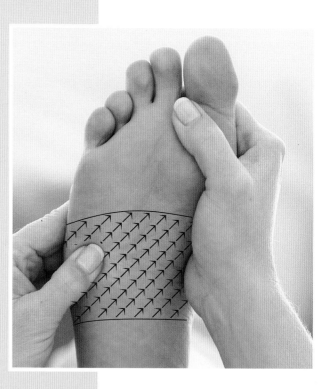

Liver
The liver reflex is only on the right foot. Holding the foot with your left hand, creep across the reflex area with your right thumb. Work from the medial to the lateral side at the angle shown (above). Switch hands and work back across the area in the opposite direction (right).

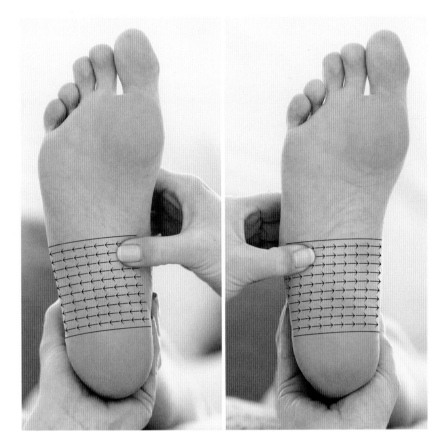

Intestines

Support the right foot with your left hand. Using your right thumb, work over the area below the waist line (see page 10) down to the base of the foot with your right thumb, moving in straight lines from the medial to the lateral side (far left). Change hands and use your left thumb to work back from the lateral to the medial side (left). Then, work the left foot starting with your left thumb.

Stomach

This reflex is only on the left foot, between the waist and diaphragm lines (see page 10). Supporting the left foot with your right hand, work over the area with your left thumb. Work from the medial to the lateral side of the foot (right), then switch hands and work back with your right thumb (far right).

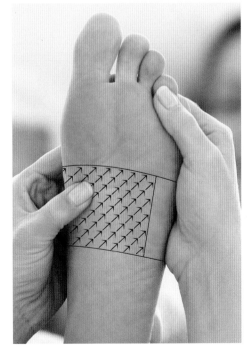

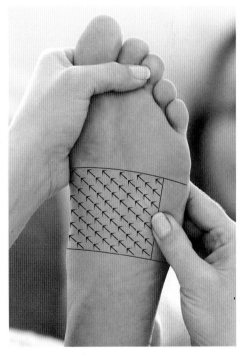

Treating painful periods

Your womb contracts and relaxes regularly throughout the month, but in the week before your period the contractions become stronger to eliminate the lining of the womb. Menstruation may be painful when the contractions are too strong or when there is too much of the hormone-like substance called prostaglandin in the body. Reflexology can bring rapid relief from period pain and will soon make you feel better, particularly if you have severe cramping. The most important reflexes to work are those relating to the reproductive system. Constipation can make matters worse as a congested bowel puts pressure on the uterus, so be particularly careful with your diet the week before a period. Gentle exercise, such as yoga, walking and swimming, help by increasing blood circulation in the pelvic region.

Areas to work
- Uterus
- Ovaries
- Fallopian tubes

Why not try?

The herb dong quai – it has been used for centuries as a tonic to the womb. Dong quai helps normal functioning of the womb by reducing the severity of the contractions and by improving blood circulation. Dong quai is also a natural anti-inflammatory, which helps reduce the pain of difficult menstruation.

Self-help

Try these simple tips to ease period pain.

- Some women find that vitamin B6 reduces the intensity of period pains significantly.

- Magnesium acts as a muscle relaxant and it has been shown to have a beneficial effect on painful periods and low back pain.

- Sipping chamomile tea can ease pain and tension and raspberry leaf tea helps to reduce bloating.

- Relaxing in a warm bath with five drops of chamomile, marjoram or cypress oil in the water helps soothe abdominal cramps.

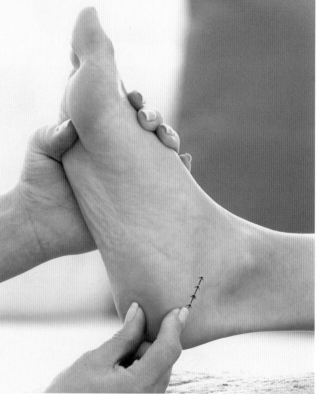

Uterus
Hold the right foot with your left hand. The reflex point for the uterus is between the heel and the ankle bone on the medial side, so work across this area from the tip of the heel with your right index finger. Change hands to work the left foot.

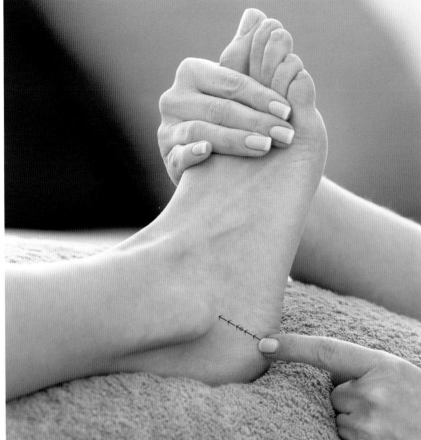

Ovaries

Hold the right foot with your right hand. The reflex point for the ovaries is between the heel and the ankle bone on the lateral side of the foot, so use your left index finger to creep from the tip of the heel to the ankle bone. Change hands to work the left foot.

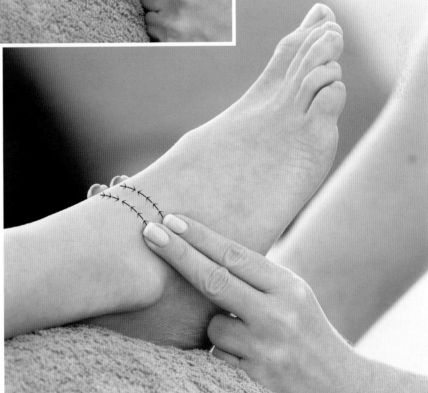

Fallopian tubes

Using both thumbs, press into the sole of the right foot. As you do this, creep across the top of the foot with the index and third fingers of both hands. Repeat two or three times, then change hands to work the left foot.

Treating headaches

Headaches can be a problem at any age, not just during the teenage years. This is the time, however, when many young women first start getting headaches, perhaps linked to PMT or anxieties about school and exams. There are many causes, including dehydration, colds and flu, low blood sugar, stress, tiredness and eye strain. Reflexology can bring immediate relief from headaches and can also be used to treat the cause if they are recurrent for a particular reason.

Try to avoid taking aspirin, which can irritate the stomach, and don't drink coffee while you have a headache as it will dehydrate you even more. If you find you get headaches when working at your desk or at your computer, try not to work more than two hours at a stretch. Then get up and walk around the room. Stretch your arms above your head and rotate your wrists. Make the time for a glass of fruit juice or herbal tea before returning to work.

Areas to work

- Neck and head
- Upper spine
- Metatarsal kneading
- Diaphragm relax

Why not try?

A cold compress – it can be very soothing. Put six ice cubes in a small jug of water and add five drops of rose, geranium or chamomile essential oil. Soak some cotton wool or a soft flannel in this solution, then lie down and place the compress on your forehead and temples. Relax for at least ten minutes.

Neck and head

This helps to relax all areas from the back of the neck to the top of the head. Hold the right foot with your left hand. Using your right thumb, creep up the underside of the big toe, second and third toes in turn. Change hands to work the left foot.

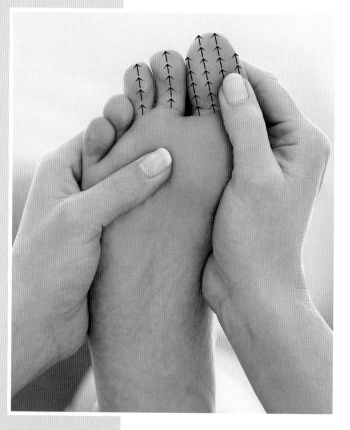

Self-help

- Headaches can be a sign of eye strain so go to your optician for an eye check.

- Drink plenty of water to flush out your system and take a teaspoon of honey to restore your blood sugar level.

- Relax in a warm bath. Add five drops of lavender, peppermint or marjoram essential oil to the water.

- If you feel sick when you have a headache, try sipping a cup of peppermint tea.

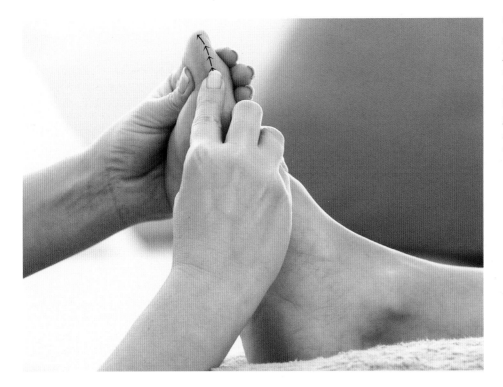

Upper spine
Hold the right foot with your left hand. With your right thumb, creep up the medial side of the foot from the waist line (see page 10) to the top of the big toe. Change hands to work the left foot.

Now relax

These are particularly beneficial treatments for anyone suffering from stress or stress-related conditions such as headaches. They slow respiration and help you feel calm and relaxed, leaving all your tensions behind. For more relaxation techniques see pages 116–17.

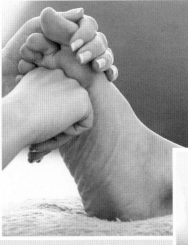

Metatarsal kneading
Push your right fist into the sole of the right foot. At the same time, squeeze the top of the foot with your left hand, making an action rather like kneading dough. Change hands to work the left foot.

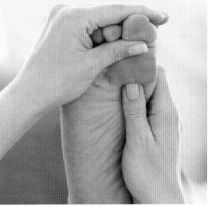

Diaphragm relax
Hold the top of the right foot with your left hand. Place your right thumb on the start of the diaphragm line (see p. 10). Press your thumb into the foot and work along the diaphragm line to the lateral edge. As you do this, bend the top of the foot over onto your left thumb. Change hands to treat the left foot.

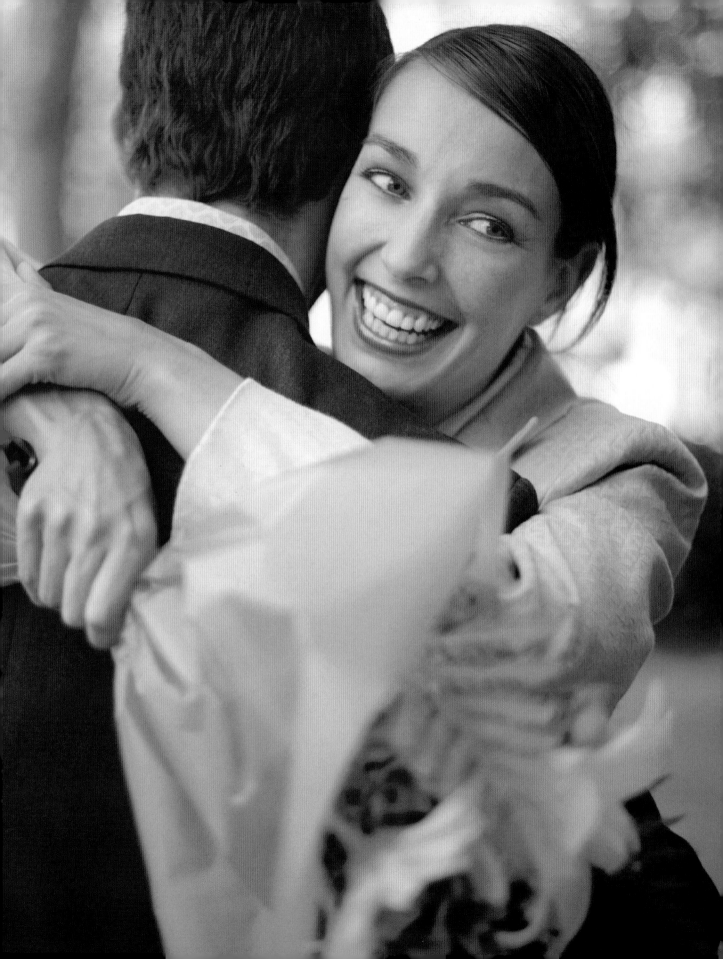

Reflexology and fertility

If you and your partner are in good health before you begin trying to conceive you will give your baby the best possible start in life. It is as – if not even more – important to improve your lifestyle and diet at this time as when you are pregnant, so make sure you eat well, stop smoking and cut right down on alcohol. Try to correct any vitamin and mineral deficiencies and avoid toxins as far as you can. If you have been taking the contraceptive pill, stop and use barrier methods such as condoms and diaphragms for the months prior to trying to conceive.

You can benefit enormously from reflexology during the preconceptual stage. Working on each other's feet at least three times a week will balance the hormonal system, improve nerve and blood supply to the entire body and encourage the body to detoxify. This creates the best possible environment for conception.

You will also find that just making time to give each other a reflexology treatment brings you closer together as a couple and encourages ideal circumstances for the creation of a new life.

Preparing for pregnancy

It's worth thinking ahead to be sure you are in peak condition for pregnancy. Your partner's health is just as important. It takes at least three months for sperm cells to mature, ready to be ejaculated so the healthier he is, the better the quality of his sperm.

Eat well

Keep a careful check on your diet. Avoid additives, preservatives and chemicals – artificial sweeteners in particular are bad for you. Reduce your intake of caffeine and alcohol. Avoid sugar both on its own and in foods – sugar whether brown or white is addictive and has no food value whatsoever. Eat oily fish, seeds and nuts to increase your intake of essential fatty acids (EFAs), vital for the making and repairing of cells. EFAs also encourage the production of healthy prostaglandins, which support body functions such as heart rate, blood pressure and blood clotting as well as fertility and conception.

• Make sure you eat plenty of fruit and vegetables – at least five servings a day, preferably more.

• Eat complex carbohydrates – wholegrains, such as brown rice, oats and wholemeal bread.

• Choose organic foods as often as you can afford.

• Include phyto-oestrogens (plant oestrogens), such as lentils, chickpeas and soya products, in your diet.

• Eat oily foods including fish, nuts, seeds and oils. Current advice for women who are pregnant or planning to conceive is to eat oily fish no more than twice a week because of possible risks from pollutants and chemicals.

Your supplement plan

Take a good multivitamin and mineral supplement designed for pregnancy (it must contain 400 micrograms of folic acid), plus the following nutrients at these dosages. Your partner should follow the same vitamin/supplement plan.

NAME	AMOUNT
Folic acid (from vitamin and mineral supplement)	400 micrograms per day
Vitamin B12	20 micrograms per day
Zinc citrate	30 milligrams per day
Selenium	100 micrograms per day
Vitamin E	300 micrograms per day
Linseed (flaxseed oil)	1000 milligrams per day
Vitamin C	1000 milligrams per day

Watch your weight

Being female and overweight can contribute to difficulties in conceiving. Oestrogen is held in our fat cells and an excess of fat means an excess of oestrogen, which can be a problem. Excess weight can also lead to menstrual and ovulation difficulties. Men need to be careful, too, as men who are overweight are more likely to produce low-quality sperm.

Being female and underweight or having a history of anorexia can stop menstruation altogether. When body weight becomes too low, the reproductive system ceases to produce a monthly cycle. A weak, poorly nourished body cannot provide the right environment for conception. The body never knows whether it is in the process of 'feast or famine' and so protects itself by shutting down fertility.

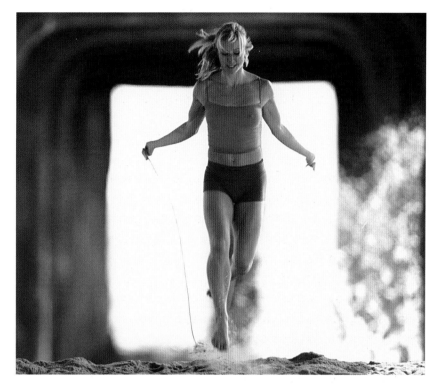

Fit for the birth
The fitter you are before conceiving, the better you will be able to cope with both pregnancy and childbirth.

Folic acid

The most important supplement when preparing for pregnancy is folic acid. It is believed to ensure that a baby reaches a healthy birth weight and it protects against DNA malfunctioning, reducing the risk of spina bifida. Folic acid is particularly important for women who have previously experienced a miscarriage. To boost your levels, eat foods that are rich in folic acid, such as beans, lentils, granary bread and green leafy vegetables, in the months before conception, and start taking a supplement. Continue taking folic acid for the first three months of pregnancy. If you don't like taking tablets folic acid is available in a drink form.

Stop smoking and drinking

If you or your partner are smokers, stop well before you start trying to conceive. It can cause infertility and sperm problems and has also been linked to premature births. Alcohol can reduce fertility, too, and increases the risk of miscarriage. Smoking is one of the worst things you can do for your future baby's health.

Infertility

Difficulty in conceiving a child is an increasing problem in the Western
world and as many as one in six couples suffer from some degree of
infertility. A couple is considered to be infertile if they haven't conceived
after having unprotected intercourse for a year. Many of these couples,
however, are only subfertile – they have low fertility – and are likely to
conceive with another year of trying.

If you have problems conceiving a child you may have feelings of
panic, frustration and despair. Some women become so psychologically
affected by their inability to conceive that they suffer severe depression,
which only adds to the problem. But a diagnosis of infertility does not
necessarily mean that you will always be infertile. There are many reasons
for fertility problems, including hormonal imbalances, sexually transmitted
disease, nutritional deficiencies and damage to the reproductive organs
due to previous infections such as pelvic inflammatory disease, but many
of these can be treated.

Some people think that long-term use of the contraceptive pill may
affect a woman's ability to conceive, but doctors now believe this is not
the case. It may, however, take a few months for the normal menstrual
cycle to resume after stopping the pill or other contraceptive devices,
such as implants.

When aiming to find a solution to infertility it is vital to realize the
importance of treating the whole body. We are not just a variety of body
parts – every organ and part of the body interacts. Using reflexology
as an aid to good health will encourage fertility as well as establish an
overall sense of well-being.

How reflexology can help

Reflexology seems to stimulate and stabilize the whole hormonal system,
encouraging the body to establish a normal cycle, and it also has a
calming effect on the body, mind and spirit. Hormones are like chemical
messengers that are carried in the bloodstream – the word hormone
comes from a Greek word meaning to urge on. Reflexology does just
this – it urges the body to work efficiently. Hormones in harmony are
essential for reproduction and this balance can be achieved by regular
reflexology treatment sessions, working particularly on the endocrine and
reproductive systems.

Women ovulate from alternate ovaries each month and you will find
that reflex points in your feet identify which ovary is active during your

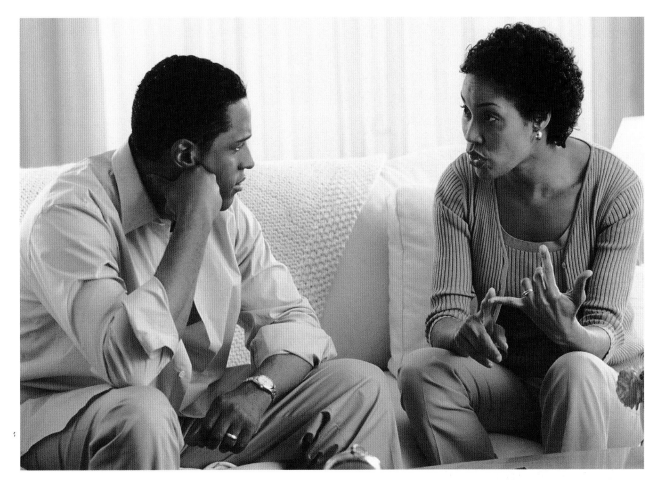

cycle – the reflex point linked to the ovulating ovary will be extremely sensitive when reflexology pressure is applied. This gives you an excellent guide as to what is going on in your body, and shows you when is the best time to have intercourse.

Is it me or my partner?

When a couple is infertile it may be to do with the woman's problems, the man's or a combination of the two – for example, some women have an allergic reaction to their partner's sperm. Investigation of the female system is more complex than that of the male, however, so the first check should be that the male partner is producing sufficient normal healthy sperm. A man releases approximately 20 million sperm at each ejaculation, 50 per cent of which need to be actively moving. The sperm that penetrates the egg needs to have sufficient motility (mobility) to burrow through the membrane surrounding the female egg cell.

In the last fifty years the average sperm count has decreased in Western countries by 40 per cent and some men are found to have

Talk about it

If you are having problems conceiving a child, it always helps to talk about your worries. If you decide to see a counsellor or a fertility expert, it is important that you attend as a couple.

sperm with low motility. A low sperm count is not necessarily a problem, as such large amounts of sperm are produced, but the quality and motility of the sperm do matter. It is still possible to conceive with a low sperm count, however, and the next step is to improve your fertility.

Some of the causes of reduced fertility

• Alcohol can reduce your fertility by half; heavy drinking binges are quite disastrous for your reproductive system. A glass of wine a day is acceptable but more will lessen your ability to conceive.

• Smoking can damage the sperm's ability to fertilize the egg and affects blood supply to the ovaries and uterus in women. It can also cause hormone imbalances and reduce the chances of the embryo implanting.

• Mobile phones send destructive rays through the delicate areas of the brain, affecting the pituitary gland. This has an impact on fertility as well as other hormonal functions. Only use your mobile phone, therefore, when absolutely necessary.

• Xenoestrogens are environmental pollutants from products such as plastics and pesticides that we are bombarded with today. These pesticides/chemicals eventually drain through the earth and into our water supply. No filtering system can stop this invasion of xenoestrogens. Hormonal pollutants also come from the many women taking the contraceptive pill, hormone replacement therapy and infertility drugs. These hormones are expelled during urination, so again become a part of our water supply.

• Electromagnetic radiation (EMR) may affect fertility so avoid using electric blankets, microwave ovens and sunbeds in the months prior to conceiving and during the first three months of pregnancy.

• Chemicals in the workplace can affect reproductive health so investigate any possible problems. You may need to avoid certain substances for a short while.

• Mineral deficiencies in the body are well known to cause reduced fertility as well as problems in pregnancy and a baby's failure to thrive. You might want to consider having a hair analysis test to check your levels of minerals and toxic metals.

Supplements to boost fertility

Because of the way our food is produced today many people are deficient in the vitamins that are essential for producing the genetic material of the next generation.

• Zinc is essential for the health and functioning of our thyroid gland. A low thyroid function can affect fertility. Vegetables and fruit used to be grown in zinc-rich soil, but with modern farming methods much of this has been destroyed and our supplies of this mineral may be low. Zinc is also necessary to use the reproductive hormones, oestrogen and progesterone, efficiently. Zinc deficiency can cause chromosome changes in both partners, leading to infertility and increased risk of miscarriage. Zinc is found in high concentrations in the sperm and adequate levels are needed to make the outer layer and the tail.

• Selenium is an important antioxidant, which helps to protect your body from free radicals. Selenium can prevent chromosome breakdown and DNA damage, which are known to be a cause of miscarriage and birth defects. Selenium is also needed for healthy sperm formation so it is important that both you and your partner take this supplement.

• Vitamin C is an anti-inflammatory – inflammation in the fallopian tubes can prevent conception. Vitamin C also helps make sperm more active.

• The B vitamins help to maintain the health of our nervous system. If you are jittery and jumpy and suffer from nervous stress from time to time you may well be deficient in B vitamins. Vitamin B6 and magnesium are necessary for the pituitary gland to secrete two valuable hormones – follicle stimulating hormone and the luteinizing hormone.

Herbal remedies

Provided you are not in the process of taking medically prescribed drugs to help your infertility you might like to try some herbal remedies. Never at any time combine herbal remedies with medical drugs for infertility.

• Agnus castus is a hormone-balancing hormone. Take daily for at least three months.

• Saw palmetto acts like a tonic, toning and strengthening the male reproductive system. Your partner should take it daily for three months.

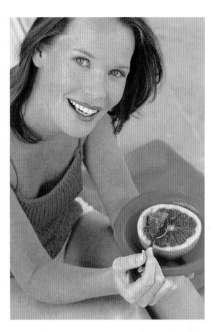

Get fresh
Fresh, unprocessed food contains the maximum number of vitamins and nutrients. Choose organically grown fruit and vegetables as often as you can.

Stress and fertility

Stress can affect your ability to conceive. When the body is stressed the adrenal glands, which are little caps that sit on top of the kidneys, release adrenalin. Adrenalin is the hormone that triggers the flee, fight and fright reactions in the body and has widespread effects on circulation, the muscles and sugar metabolism. When adrenalin is released, the action of the heart and the body's metabolic rate is increased. At the same time, the blood and nerve supply to the bladder, intestines, reproductive system and immune support is decreased.

Today's high-speed world strains our body and emotions. So many of us are trying to do too much in too little time, as we battle with work problems, tensions in the home, financial worries and so on. Many people have a very high adrenalin output most of the time, causing the body to believe it is about to run for its life, fight to survive, or face a terrifying situation – not the right environment for conception. The adrenal glands start producing hormones that dampen down the reproductive system in an attempt to protect the body against conception if it believes a life-threatening event is imminent.

Try to reduce stress levels by exercising regularly to reduce tension and maybe taking up something calming such as yoga or meditation. Consider counselling if stress becomes severe.

Some time off can help too. When we go on holiday, perhaps in a warm climate, with a couple of weeks to relax, enjoy the sunshine, swim and live closer to nature, we become de-stressed. As we relax, adrenal activity returns to normal and research has found that sunlight increases testosterone levels, the hormone that stimulates sexual desire. It also stimulates the pituitary gland, which stimulates the hormones controlling the reproductive system. So, provided your fertile period comes at the right time, you may be more likely to conceive while on holiday.

Easing stress with reflexology

The correct functioning of the reproductive system of both men and women is very susceptible to stress and tension so reflexology can be of great benefit in this situation. In women, menstruation can stop completely if stress levels are too high, and men who are over-stressed may find it almost impossible to maintain an erection. I have known many couples, who have had difficulty in conceiving a child, succeed after regular treatment by a reflexologist, provided there is no medical problem that prevents pregnancy. It is usually important for both partners to be treated and treatment may take several months.

Good news

When the great moment arrives and you find out you are pregnant, you will be all the happier, knowing you have prepared your body as well as you can for what is to come.

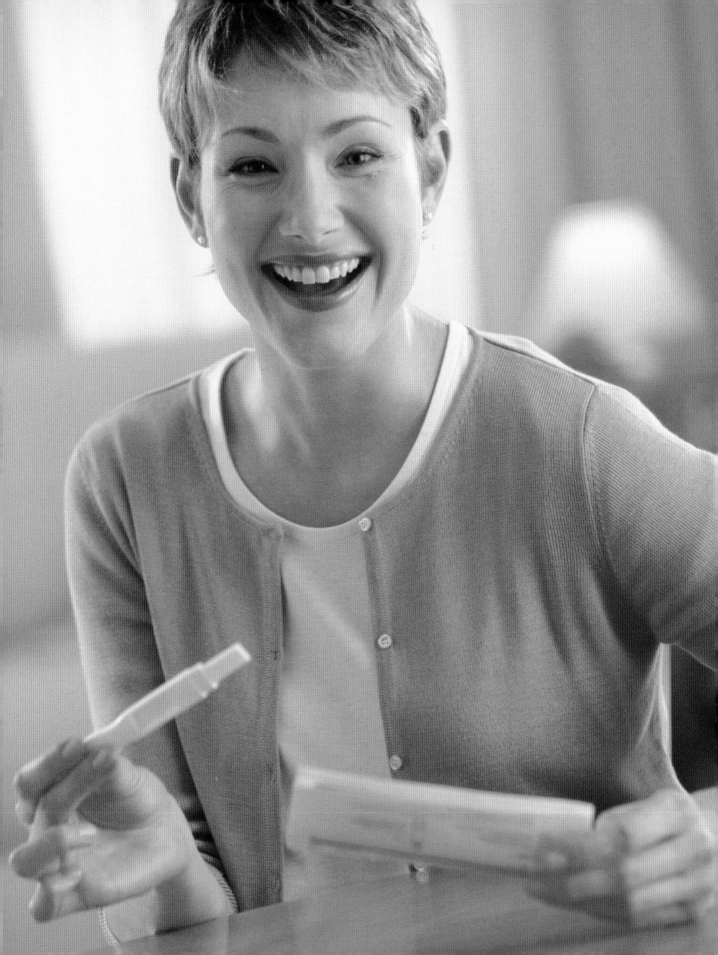

Treatments to boost fertility and aid conception

Enhance your chances of conceiving with regular reflexology treatment to balance your hormones and bring your body into peak condition. Treatment helps you focus on your body and relieves stress and tension. Take it in turns to treat each other a few times a week, but for best results you may like to see a professional reflexologist over a period of three or four months.

Areas to work

- Pituitary
- Thyroid (plantar and dorsal)
- Uterus
- Ovaries
- Fallopian tubes
- Spinal stimulation point

Why not try?

Giving up caffeine – some research has shown that drinking only one cup of coffee a day reduces your chances of conceiving. Remember, there is caffeine in tea, cola drinks and chocolate as well as coffee.

Self-help

You owe it to your baby to be in the best possible health before conceiving.

- Stop smoking. This applies to both you and your partner. Avoid exposure to passive smoking as far as possible.

- Reduce or cut out alcohol and don't take any recreational drugs.

- Eat fresh, wholesome foods, including plenty of fruit and vegetables. Buy organic if you can afford it.

- Take regular exercise and think about starting meditation as a way of relaxing and improving your stress levels.

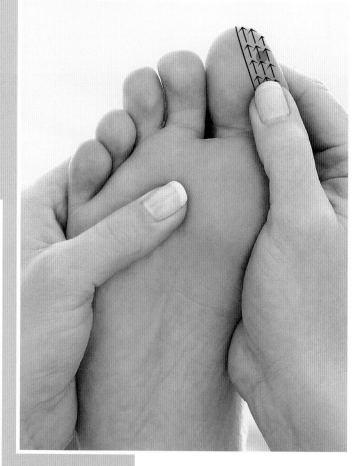

Pituitary
Hold the right foot with your left hand. Starting at the base, creep up the big toe with your right thumb. Change hands to work the left foot.

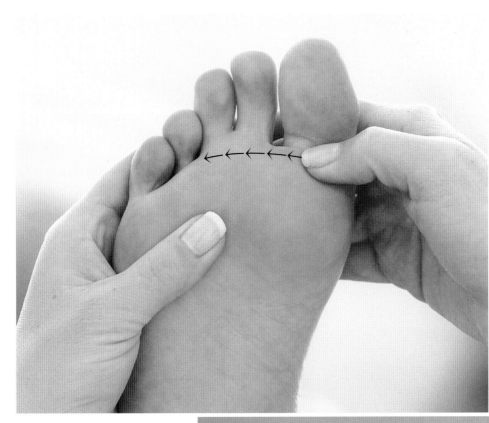

Thyroid (plantar)

Hold the right foot with your left hand. Use your right thumb to creep along the bases of the first three toes. Repeat three times. Change hands to treat the left foot.

Thyroid (dorsal)

Support the right foot with your left fist. With your right index finger, creep along the base of the first three toes. Repeat three times. Change hands to treat the left foot.

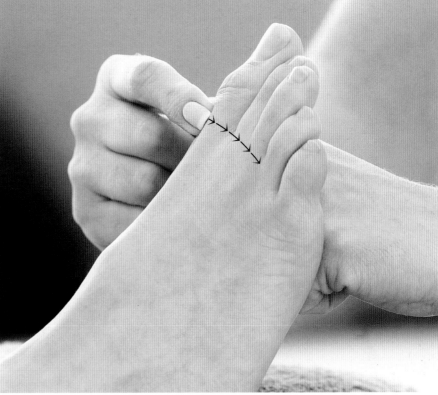

Uterus

Hold the right foot with your left hand. The reflex point for the uterus is between the heel and the ankle bone on the medial side, so work across this area from the tip of the heel with your right index finger. Change hands to work the left foot.

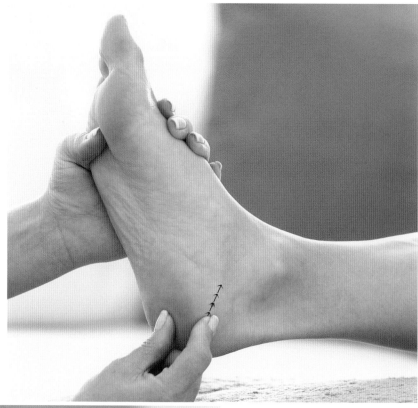

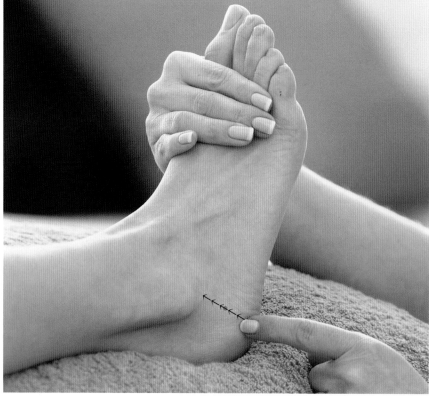

Ovaries

Hold the right foot with your right hand. The reflex point for the ovaries is between the heel and the ankle bone on the lateral side of the foot, so use your left index finger to creep from the tip of the heel to the ankle bone. Change hands to work the left foot. (This is also the reflex for the testes in men.)

Fallopian tubes

Using both thumbs, press into the sole of the right foot. As you do this, creep across the top of the foot with the index and third fingers of both hands. Repeat two or three times. Change hands to work the left foot. (This is also the reflex point for the vas deferens in men.)

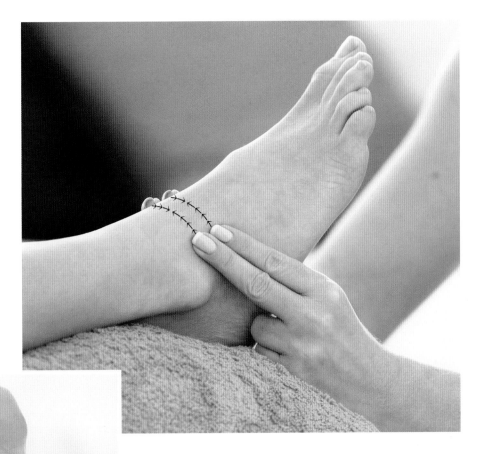

Spinal stimulation point

Support the right foot in your left hand. Find the spinal stimulation point in the middle of the medial side of the foot and using your right thumb, make five or six rotations. Change hands to work the left foot. This reflex point energizes the whole spinal area.

It takes two to conceive

The prospective father will benefit from reflexology treatment too. These are the main areas to work on in addition to a complete treatment:

- Pituitary (see page 58)
- Thyroid (see page 59)
- Testes (see ovaries, page 60)
- Vas deferens (see fallopian tubes, page 61)
- Spinal stimulation point (see page 61)

Miscarriage

Suffering a miscarriage can be a profoundly distressing experience for a woman and her partner. It is a huge physical and emotional shock that most people are just not prepared for. One in four pregnancies end in a miscarriage, and chromosomal abnormalities are thought to be responsible in 50 per cent of miscarriages. A miscarriage is the spontaneous loss of a foetus before the 24th week of pregnancy. After 24 weeks the loss of a baby is a stillbirth.

When recovering from the emotional and physical effects of a miscarriage, I recommend that you and your partner give each other reflexology on a weekly basis. Treatment will bring about a feeling of relaxation and peace and help to build up the woman's confidence in her ability to conceive and carry a healthy baby to full term.

Many women don't want to think about conceiving again for at least four months, but, when you do feel ready, you need to be in the best

Supporting each other
You will need plenty of support after a miscarriage. It can be hard to come to terms with your loss and you may find counselling helpful.

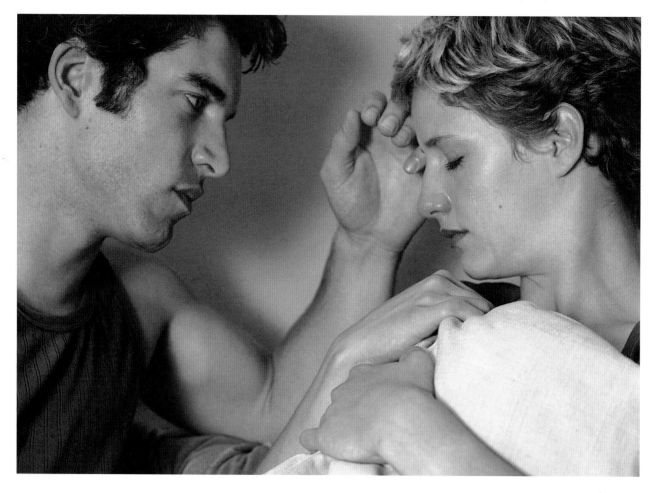

possible health and minimize the risk of miscarrying again by paying strict attention to lifestyle changes and diet. Follow the advice on preconceptual health at the beginning of this chapter with great care and pay particular attention to the supplement suggestions below. For example, researchers have found that women who miscarry have low levels of selenium in their blood compared to women who don't miscarry.

Reduce your intake of saturated fats, which are abundant in dairy products. Both red meat and dairy produce contain arachidonic acid, which encourages the production of PGE2, a prostaglandin that leads to abnormal blood flow and blood clotting. When you are trying to prevent a miscarriage the aim is to reduce any abnormal blood clotting.

Herbal remedies

There are three herbs that can be very beneficial in the prevention of miscarriage and they should be taken during the four-month preconceptual period.

• Agnus castus can be a great help for women after a miscarriage. It is said to stimulate the function of the pituitary gland, which controls and balances our hormones by producing the luteinizing hormone.

• Blue cohosh is another important herb for the reproductive system. It tones and strengthens the whole system and is particularly useful for prevention of miscarriages. It is believed to be a tonic for the womb and the whole of the reproductive system.

• False unicorn root is usually used in combination with the other herbs above in order to help prevent a miscarriage.

Supplements to take after a miscarriage

The following supplements are particularly helpful for women who have suffered miscarriages. Take these for three to four months.

• Multivitamin
• Folic acid
• Vitamin E
• Zinc
• Selenium
• Essential fatty acids

Treatments to aid recovery from miscarriage

The miscarriage of a longed-for baby is always distressing, whatever the cause, and you need time to recover emotionally as well as physically. It can also take several months for the normal menstrual cycle to be restored after a miscarriage. Use reflexology to help re-balance the body and establish the cycle once more. Most women also find that reflexology helps them recover from the emotional trauma of miscarriage, healing the spirit as well as the body.

Areas to work

- Pituitary
- Thyroid (plantar and dorsal)
- Spinal stimulation point
- Uterus
- Ovaries

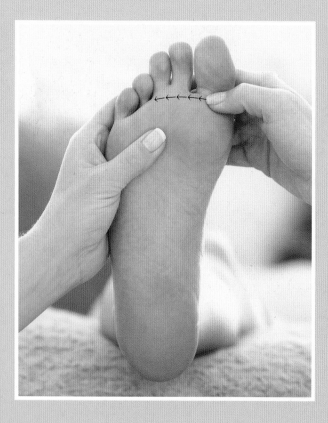

Pituitary

Hold the right foot with your left hand. Starting at the base, creep up the big toe with your right thumb. Change hands to work the left foot.

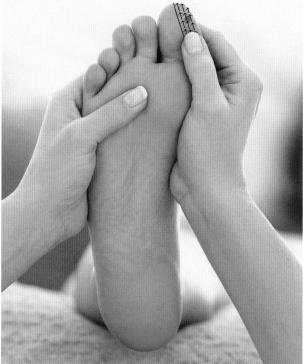

Thyroid (plantar)

Hold the right foot with your left hand. Use your right thumb to creep along the bases of the first three toes. Repeat three times. Change hands to treat the left foot.

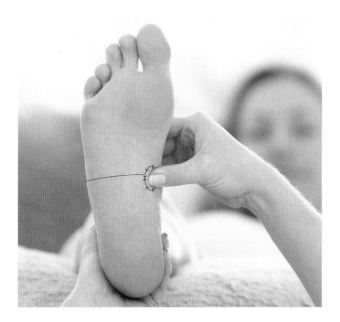

Spinal stimulation point

Support the right foot in your left hand. Find the spinal stimulation point in the middle of the medial side of the foot and using your right thumb, make five or six rotations. Change hands to work the left foot. This reflex point energizes the whole spinal area.

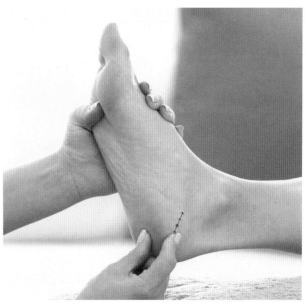

Uterus

Hold the right foot with your left hand. The reflex point for the uterus is between the heel and the ankle bone on the medial side, so work across this area from the tip of the heel with your right index finger. Change hands to work the left foot.

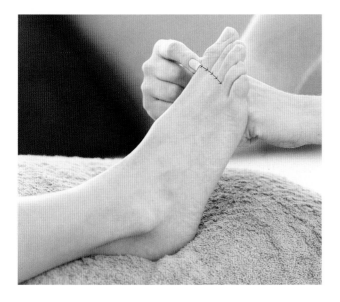

Thyroid (dorsal)

Support the right foot with your left fist. With your right index finger, creep along the base of the first three toes. Repeat three times. Change hands to treat the left foot.

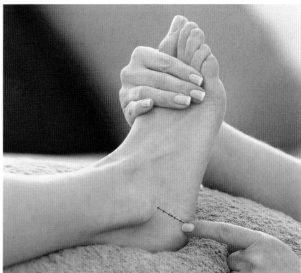

Ovaries

Hold the right foot with your right hand. The reflex point for the ovaries is between the heel and the ankle bone on the lateral side, so use your left index finger to creep from the tip of the heel to the ankle bone. Change hands to work the left foot.

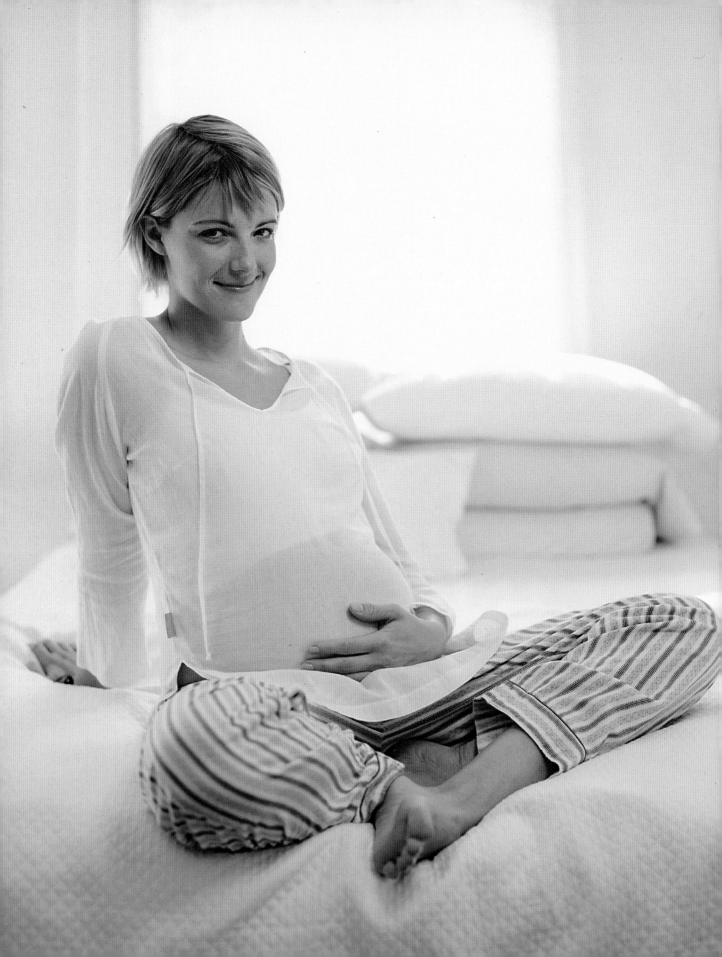

Reflexology during pregnancy

At no other time in your life is it more vital to look after yourself than from the moment you find out you are pregnant. It is best to pay special attention to your health before you even start trying to conceive because the human body needs huge reserves of energy to stabilize a pregnancy and develop a new life. The better your own and your partner's health, the better start you give your baby.

Your baby's life begins with a single cell – one of your eggs fused with one of your partner's sperm. From this tiny cell, which is even smaller than the full stop at the end of this paragraph, come the building blocks necessary to control the genetic material for the growth and development of a baby. Over the nine months of pregnancy, your body needs plenty of energy to nurture your growing baby in the womb and to develop a supply of milk for the early months of the infant's life.

Reflexology is a safe and beneficial therapy for use at this time of physical and psychological adjustment, but during the first three months of pregnancy it is best to go to a qualified practitioner for treatment. Always tell anyone giving you reflexology that you are pregnant.

A healthy pregnancy

Pregnancy is not an illness. A woman's body was designed for giving birth and nurturing her young, and for many women, childbirth is one of life's most amazing emotional and physical experiences. Get yourself off to a good start by being extra careful about what you eat and drink, following the tips suggested below.

If you do have any health problems, though, such as indigestion or back pain, reflexology is a safe and effective complementary therapy that can be used during your pregnancy to relieve all kinds of discomforts. It also helps to prepare your body for the delivery. You may like to ask the person who has treated you while you are pregnant to be with you during the birth, so she can work on some special reflex points in the feet during your labour.

Eating well

Food cravings may be your body's way of telling you it needs certain nutrients or foods, but do try to deal with these sensibly. If you crave sweet foods, eat dried apricots and raisins rather than a chocolate bar. If you crave salty foods, maybe a few pickles would help, whereas packets of salty crisps would not be good for you. Too much salt retains fluid in the tissues of the body, places an undue strain on the circulation and increases your blood pressure.

If constipation is troubling you, try to increase dietary fibre by eating more wholegrains and vegetables. Some olive oil on your salads helps to prevent your bowel contents becoming too dry or you could take a couple of teaspoons

No need to eat for two
A good diet is essential during pregnancy, but you don't need to eat for two as people used to believe. Most women will only need an extra few hundred calories a day. Just eat good-quality fresh foods, with plenty of fruit and vegetables.

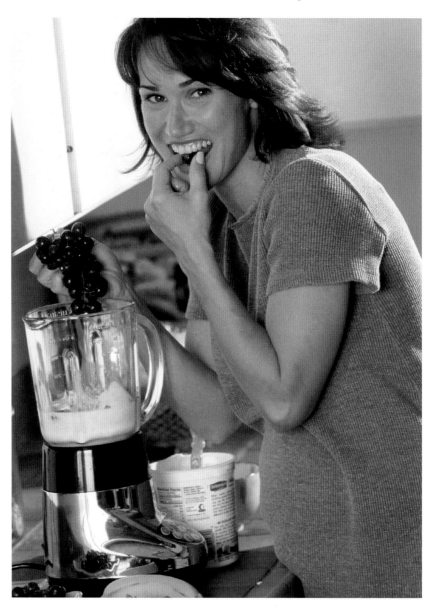

of oil each day. Make sure that you drink plenty of fluids so that the fibre in your diet swells up in the bowel, encouraging an easier evacuation of your waste products.

Supplements

Our bodies need iron to make red blood cells, which carry oxygen to all parts of the body. During pregnancy you need extra iron for the increased amount of blood in your body. Make sure that you eat plenty of iron-rich foods, such as green vegetables, broccoli, spinach and red meat; nuts and seeds such as sunflower and pumpkin are also recommended. All mothers used to be prescribed iron supplements whether or not they were anaemic, but doctors now prefer to recommend supplements only if needed. Too much iron is thought to be bad for you and also increases the risk of constipation.

Your body also needs magnesium to help make bone, protein and fatty acids. It also helps to relax the muscles of the womb and is a natural tranquilliser. If you are going through a stressful period in your life, try taking 200 milligrams of magnesium a day, which is the optimum dose. You may find that taking this mineral at night helps you rest, particularly if your expanding uterus makes it difficult for you to get comfortable and disturbs your sleep patterns.

Research tells us that a deficiency in folic acid increases the risk of having a baby with neural tube defects such as spina bifida. Doctors recommend that you take folic acid as soon as you start trying to conceive and continue until the end of the third month of pregnancy (see page 51). At this stage of your pregnancy the baby's neural tube, or spinal cord as it is sometimes referred to, will be properly formed.

Alcohol and cigarettes

It is best to avoid alcohol during pregnancy, particularly in the early weeks when the highest rate of cell division takes place and all the baby's major organs are being formed. Alcohol is a toxin and if any of these toxins pass through the placental wall they could affect your unborn baby's brain and nervous system.

Smoking causes all manner of serious diseases and during pregnancy it affects the unborn child as well as the mother. Nicotine is a stimulant and causes the fetal heart rate to accelerate. The hundreds of chemicals in tobacco have a constricting effect on the arteries so as you smoke the blood supply to your baby will be compromised. Your partner should give up, too, as passive smoking can harm your unborn child, and you.

A balanced diet

You don't need special foods during pregnancy, just regular, balanced meals containing a wide range of nutrients.

• At least five servings of fresh fruit and vegetables every day, more if you can.

• Calcium-rich foods such as yogurt, milk and pasteurized cheeses.

• Proteins, such as meat, fish and well-cooked eggs. Eat pulses if you are vegetarian.

• Carbohydrates such as wholegrain cereals and bread, rice and pasta.

• At least two litres of fluid a day – preferably water.

Problems in pregnancy

Some mothers sail through pregnancy, look wonderful and say that they have never felt so well in their life. The huge increase in hormonal activity often makes the skin softer and hair shiny and luxurious. There are usually few aches and pains until the seventh month, when you may suffer from backache, sometimes affecting the sciatic nerve. Some women also experience pains in the thighs as the pelvic area copes not only with the weight of a baby but also the placenta.

Many women, though, suffer minor discomforts, including morning sickness, particularly common in the early weeks of pregnancy, faintness, constipation which can cause piles, and heartburn, all of which can be treated by reflexology. There are a few more serious complications that can occur, such as pre-eclampsia, but thankfully these are rare.

Morning sickness

Despite its name, morning sickness can happen at any time of day and the main cause is low blood sugar. It usually stops after the first three months. The best cure is to eat little and often. If you feel sick first thing in the morning have some dry toast or a plain biscuit and a glass of warm water to settle your stomach before you get up. Many women find that high-carbohydrate foods help as does taking ginger, peppermint herbal teas or ginger biscuits.

Because of the difficulties encountered in the past with drugs such as thalidomide, which was prescribed for morning sickness in pregnancy, doctors are not happy about prescribing any medication for this common condition. Occasionally the sickness in early pregnancy can become so acute that the mother can become dehydrated and has to go into hospital, but this is rare.

Heartburn/gastric reflux

The usual symptom of this is a burning feeling in your chest and you may find you bring up some stomach acid into your mouth. One of the causes is your expanding uterus pressing up into the abdominal areas, but it is also due to the hormones released during pregnancy that relax the valve at the entrance to your stomach. This prevents it from completely closing, allowing stomach acid to escape.

Eat little and often and try not to eat late in the evening when the heartburn is likely to get worse. It may help to sleep slightly propped up, using pillows for support.

Antacids may be recommended as they are reasonably safe during pregnancy, but antacids can affect the body's ability to absorb the iron content in your blood, and should only be used as a last resort because iron is so essential for both mother and baby. Rather than taking antacids, drink a glass of hot water for troublesome heartburn, or if you prefer, a peppermint tea several times a day. This simple remedy is most effective.

If you need to pick something up from the floor, bend at your knees and squat down. This will stop you compressing your stomach, which lies above the waist on the left side of your body.

Haemorrhoids

Haemorrhoids (dilated rectal veins) are common during pregnancy, as during this time the amount of blood circulating around your body increases, causing the veins to swell. Try to avoid haemorrhoids – also known as piles – by eating a fibre-rich diet and drinking plenty of water to keep your bowel movements regular and your stools soft. If you are troubled by these painful and often very itchy external veins, try taking a warm bath to ease the discomfort, and apply alternate cold and warm packs. There are many haemorrhoidal creams that will give you some relief. Once your baby is born you will probably find that the haemorrhoids disappear just as quickly as they came.

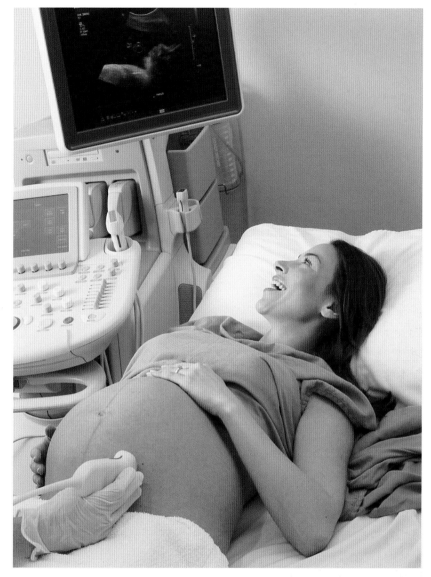

Ultrasound scans
You will have a couple of routine scans during your pregnancy to check on your baby's progress. You may also have a scan nearer full term to find out how your baby is lying or, if he is overdue, whether he is ready to be born.

Pre-eclampsia

This is a condition that can affect women after the 20th week of pregnancy. Symptoms include high blood pressure, protein in the urine and retention of fluid in the hands, feet and sometimes the face.

It is usually mild but can lead to a rare, but very serious, condition called eclampsia.

Vitamin C and E supplements are effective in preventing these symptoms and some women find that omega-3 fatty acids seem to help. It's important to rest as much as possible in order to lower blood pressure. I must stress, however, that although reflexology and the additional support of vitamin and mineral supplements help, this condition must be treated by medical experts.

Weight gain

Most experts consider a healthy weight gain during pregnancy to be not more than 15 kg (33 lb) and not less than 6 kg (13 lb). The baby accounts for about 3–4 kg (6–9 lb) of this. Putting on too much weight can increase your blood pressure and leave you several kilos heavier after the birth than you were before you became pregnant. Most women put on only a little weight during the first three months, but find weight gain speeds up around the fourth month and tails off again by about eight months. However, the amount of weight gained differs from woman to woman and pregnancy to pregnancy and you should never try to diet during pregnancy. If you feel you are gaining too much, check with your midwife and consider asking for dietary advice.

Extra fat is stored on the mother's buttocks and hips for protection of her abdominal areas. The fat store is also nature's way of ensuring that extra calories are available for mother and baby just in case food is in short supply – less likely in the West today, but something that could happen in other lands and at other times.

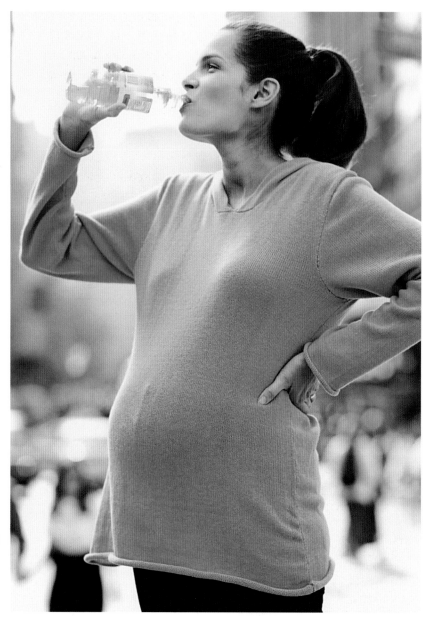

Keep drinking
Drink plenty – at least two litres of fluid a day – to keep your body hydrated. Milk and fruit juice are fine, but water is best.

Your uterus is normally only the size of a large plum, but during the 40 weeks of pregnancy it expands to the size of a large balloon. By the time you reach term it extends to the top of your diaphragm. As your uterus enlarges, stretch marks may appear on your abdomen and buttocks. Use a moisturizing cream or baby oil and massage your abdomen and buttocks daily.

Helping your body

For centuries pregnant women have drunk raspberry leaf tea. This herb helps to strengthen the pelvic and uterine muscles and establish the flow of milk to the breasts. It is best avoided in the first three months and only taken towards the end of the pregnancy as it can overstimulate the uterus in the early months.

As your cervix is going to have to stretch to allow the head of your baby to travel through the birth canal, you may find that massaging the area between the anus, vagina and the urethral opening, which is called the perineum, with olive oil, every day, will help the vagina expand more easily. Asian women have for centuries adopted this procedure to soften the perineum gradually and allow for easier dilation, thus preventing painful tears during delivery.

Toning and strengthening

The extra weight you are carrying puts a great strain on your pelvis and hips. Try these daily toning and strengthening exercises to tighten the muscles around the pelvic floor.

• Each time you stand at the sink or visit the toilet pull in the muscles around your vagina and anus. Hold them while you count to ten, then relax.

• If you like swimming, a few gentle lengths of the pool will give your whole body good exercise with the extra benefit of your joints being completely supported by water.

• Take a short walk every day while you practise some deep breathing exercises.

Treating minor ailments

Reflexology is an ideal non-invasive therapy for dealing with the minor ailments of pregnancy. Treatment will do you good and do no harm to your growing baby.

Areas to work
Constipation and haemorrhoids
• Sigmoid colon and rectum
• Intestines

Morning sickness
• Pituitary
• Stomach

Heartburn
• Stomach
• Diaphragm relaxation

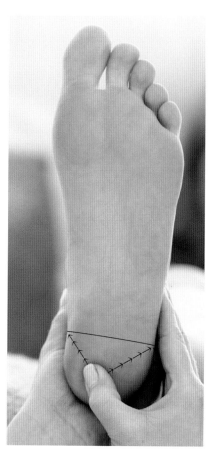

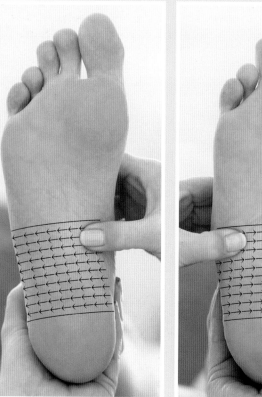

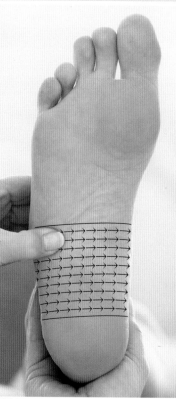

Sigmoid colon and rectum
Found only on the left foot, this V-shaped reflex lies under the pelvic line (see page 10). Holding the foot with your left hand, work up the inside fork of the reflex area with your right thumb. Change hands and work up the outside fork with the left thumb.

Intestines
Support the right foot with your left hand. Using your right thumb, work over the area below the waist line (see page 10) down to the base of the foot with your right thumb, moving in straight lines from the medial to the lateral side (far left). Change hands and use your left thumb to work back from the lateral to the medial side (left). Work the left foot starting with your left thumb.

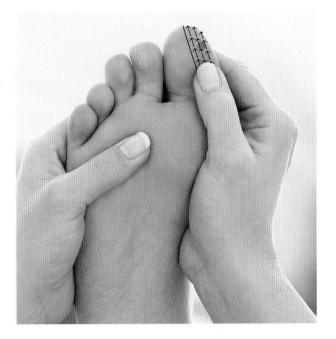

Pituitary

Hold the right foot with your left hand. Starting at the base, creep up the big toe with your right thumb. Change hands to work the left foot.

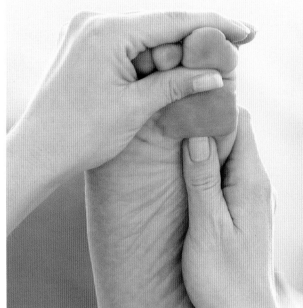

Diaphragm relax

This is a particularly beneficial treatment for anyone suffering from stress. Hold the top of the right foot with your left hand. Place your right thumb on the start of the diaphragm line (see page 10). Press your thumb into the foot and work along the diaphragm line to the lateral edge. As you do this, bend the top of the foot over onto your left thumb. Change hands to treat the left foot.

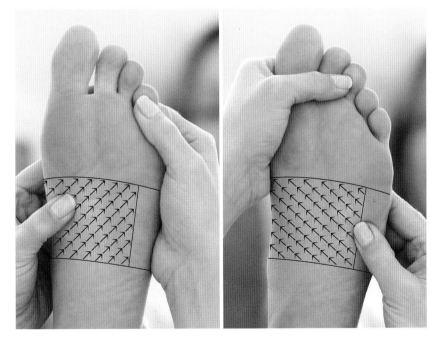

Stomach

The main stomach reflex is on the left foot, between the waist and diaphragm lines (see page 10). Supporting the left foot with your right hand, work over the area with your left thumb. Work from the medial to the lateral side of the foot, then switch hands and work back again with your right thumb.

Treating back and leg pain

Many women experience back and leg pain for the first time when pregnant, and reflexology has proved very effective in treating such symptoms. Aches and pains at this time can be caused by the action of pregnancy hormones, which soften the ligaments of the body in preparation for childbirth. This can cause strain in the lower back. Another common problem is sciatica, when the extra weight at the front of the body can put pressure on the sciatic nerve, causing pain. Sciatica that starts during pregnancy usually disappears once the baby has been born.

Areas to work

- Coccyx
- Hip and pelvis
- Spine (up)
- Spine (down)

Why not try?

A rocking chair – the gentle backwards and forwards movement is very soothing and relieves an aching back. The effects last as long as the rocking continues.

Look after your back

- Check your posture. Don't arch your back when standing and try to walk tall. Imagine you are trying to balance something on the top of your head.

- Choose a comfortable chair that supports your spine. Sit well back on the seat with your back straight and your head balanced over your hips. Don't slump.

- Try not to sit in the same position for long periods. Get up and move about the room at regular intervals.

- Make sure your bed is comfortable and supportive. Some people find that a board under the mattress helps to keep the spine straight and ease back problems.

Coccyx
Hold the top of the right foot with your right hand. Creep up the inside of the heel area with the four fingers of your left hand. Change hands to treat the left foot.

Hip and pelvis

Hold the right foot with your left hand. Using the fingers of your right hand, work the outside of the heel. Change hands to treat the left foot.

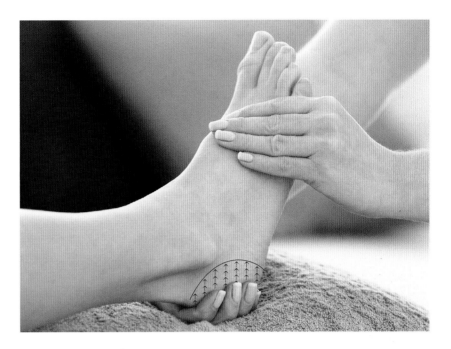

Spine (up)

Hold the right foot with your left hand. Using your right thumb, creep up the inside edge of the foot to the top of the big toe (left). Change hands to work the left foot.

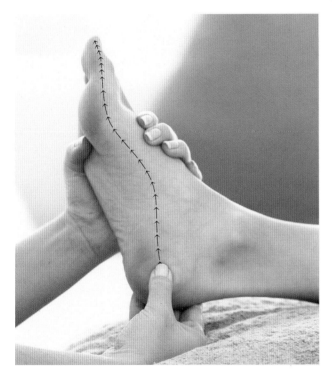

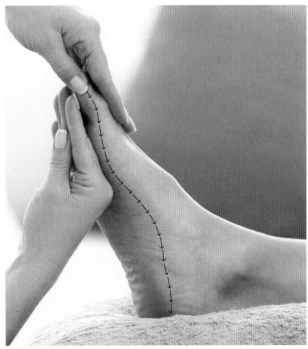

Spine (down)

Use the back of your right hand to support the sole of the right foot. Use your left thumb to creep down the inside edge of the foot (right). Move your supporting hand down as you go. Change hands to treat the left foot.

Labour and birth

Sometime around the 40th week of pregnancy your baby will become mature enough to survive in the outside world without the support of the placenta and labour will start. It is quite normal to have fears, particularly with a first pregnancy, about how your baby, contained in what seems an enormous bulge, will emerge from the small opening of the vagina. Just remember, your body is designed to cope with this.

Being born is a transition from the absolute security of the uterus to a very different world outside the mother's body. Every newborn baby needs his parents to meet his basic needs of safety, security and care in a loving, respectful and tender way.

Some mothers prefer a home birth and although this is not usually recommended in a first pregnancy, home births are becoming more popular. Other women feel more secure in a hospital environment where all the technology is available should any problems arise. During the pregnancy your doctor and midwife will help you decide what sort of birth you would prefer. For example, many women find spending at least the first part of labour in a birthing pool very relaxing. The warm water is soothing and helps ease the pain of contractions. Many maternity units now provide birthing pools, although you do need to request one in advance. You can also arrange to hire a pool for home use.

It is not unusual, say a week or so before your due date, to find you suddenly have an excess of energy. You may feel like turning out cupboards, doing lots of housework, cleaning windows and so on. This may be nature's way of encouraging you to get ready for the birth and prepare a comfortable nest for your baby.

First signs of labour

One of the first signs of the onset of labour may be the appearance of what is called the show – a plug of pinkish mucus which has sealed your cervix during pregnancy to protect against infection. You may have the show a couple of days before you start to be aware of contractions in your uterus, which have been quietly active for some days.

You may find that you also experience a tightening sensation in your uterus. Another sign of the onset of labour your waters breaking – the membranes of the amniotic sac rupture and the fluid that has cushioned your baby starts to flow out. Without warning, you may suddenly find that you are losing quite a large amount of water from your vagina. This may happen before or after you notice contractions.

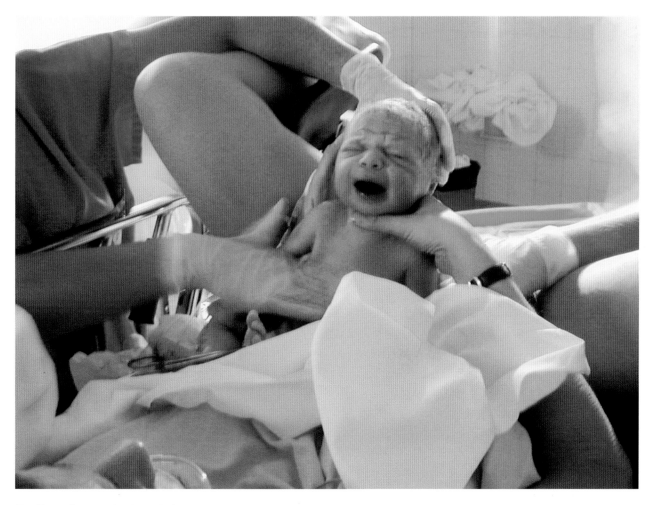

Reflexology during labour

When you start to have regular contractions, even if they are 20 minutes or so apart, it is time to contact your birthing partner and start your reflexology sessions. It is important to work on the endocrine system – the pituitary and thyroid reflexes – to encourage the hormonal demands during birth. Working the entire spinal area will help to stimulate nerve and muscle tone in the pelvic area and working the uterus will aid the contractions. Aim to treat these areas for ten minutes on each foot in every hour. You might also like to ask your birthing partner to massage the small of your back with some lavender oil. It should be quite easy to reach this area if you lie on your side.

Between reflexology sessions it is far better to keep active for as long as you can and walk around the room. Standing upright will help the contractions move your baby lower into the pelvic cavity. Women who have reflexology treatment during labour also seem to recover more quickly afterwards as the body re-balances more easily.

The moment of birth
At last – the moment you have longed for and planned for over nine months is here and you see your baby for the first time.

Coping with contractions

When the contractions are coming more frequently, are stronger and last longer it is time to go to hospital if that is where you are giving birth. If you are having a home birth, make sure that everything is ready and your birth partners and midwife are all with you.

Labours, particularly with a first baby, can last 24 hours or even longer, but second and subsequent labours are often far shorter. There is no denying that the contractions of the uterus are painful – the large horizontal and vertical uterine muscles have a terrific job to do in expelling a baby into the outside world – but it is a productive pain. Remember that with every contraction your baby is coming closer. Try as hard as you can to practise your deep breathing and breathe through a contraction instead of fighting against it.

Pain relief

During your pregnancy you will have talked with your doctor and midwife about the many safe and highly effective pain-relieving medicines that are available during labour and decided what you would prefer. These include gas and air, which you inhale, and pain-relieving injections. Some mothers prefer a spinal anaesthetic or epidural, which deadens sensation from the waist downwards and can give an almost pain-free labour. I believe, though, it is better for mother and baby if you can manage to cope without a spinal anaesthetic.

A Tens (Transcutaneous Electrical Nerve Stimulation) machine can help you to deal with labour pains naturally. This machine transmits pulses of electrical energy into your skin. These block the pain signals from reaching your brain and also promote the release of endorphins, your body's natural painkillers. You can buy or hire machines, but if you intend to use one during labour it is a good idea to practise at home in advance so you know how to use it.

Reflexology can also be a very effective form of pain relief for contractions, but treatment in this situation is best given by a trained reflexologist who is experienced in childbirth. You will also need to check with your doctors before hand that they are

Your new baby
There is nothing more fulfilling than getting to know your new baby – a wonderful little being who has developed from that minute single cell in a period of just 40 weeks.

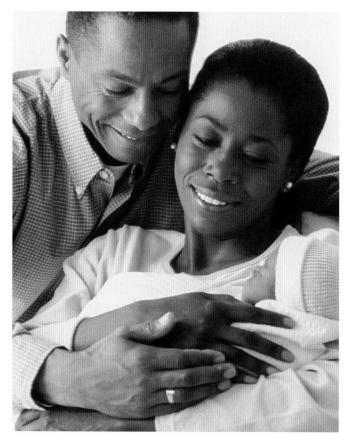

happy for you to use reflexology and be attended by a therapist,

Once your cervix is fully dilated you are ready to push your baby out. You will be encouraged to bear down with each contraction and inch by inch your baby's head will emerge. Keep doing the breathing exercises you learned in antenatal classes – they really do help. The more upright you can be the better, as the force of gravity helps move your baby down through the birth canal. If you are lying on your back it is much harder work. Once the head appears, the rest of your baby's body is usually delivered quite rapidly.

Breastfeeding

In the first days after the birth reflexology can also help establish breastfeeding, working to balance hormone levels and stimulate milk production. Here are some other tips to keep you comfortable.

• When you are breastfeeding, keep the skin of the breasts supple and well nourished with oils. If you do have cracked or sore nipples, break open a vitamin E oil capsule and rub in the oil or use some soothing lanolin cream.

• Apply the oil or cream after feeding your baby – especially after the last feed at night, so as to give the skin as much time as possible to restore itself.

• If you should get mastitis, bathe the painful areas in the breast with very hot and then very cold water. An old-fashioned but effective remedy for mastitis is to use a castor oil pack applied directly to the breast. Warm a few tablespoons of castor oil, soak a cotton wool pad in the oil and apply to the breast. Wear an old bra to keep the pad in place.

After checking that your baby's airways are clear and that he or she is breathing independently, the midwife will place your newborn son or daughter on your abdomen. Your baby has begun life in the outside world.

Breasts and breastfeeding

During your pregnancy your breasts will enlarge and the veins will become more prominent. The breasts may feel heavy and sometimes ache and feel congested. Towards the end of your pregnancy, gently massage your breast area with some lubricating oil. Start under the breast and work towards your armpit, using gentle rotating movements. This will help all the lymph nodes keep free of congestion and lessen the possibility of you getting mastitis.

It is important to wear a specially designed bra that gives you the necessary support at this time. Proper firm support will help you keep your figure by preventing undue stretching of the muscles and the skin of the upper chest. Once muscle tissue loses its original elasticity, it is virtually impossible to restore to its original shape.

Breast milk is the best possible food for a baby so if possible you will want to feed your baby yourself. Some women love breastfeeding, others get anxious and find it difficult. Do try to persevere, however. Once established, breastfeeding is easy and so convenient.

Treatment during labour

If you have been receiving reflexology through your pregnancy you might like to have some treatment during labour. It is easy to ask your reflexologist to attend if you are having a home birth, but even if you are having your baby in hospital it shouldn't be a problem. More and more hospitals are willing to be flexible about arrangements like this, but you should certainly discuss it with your medical team well in advance of the birth. If your partner has been giving you reflexology, he can continue to do so during labour. Work on each foot for ten minutes in every hour.

Areas to work

When the contractions start, work on the following:

- Pituitary
- Uterus
- Coccyx
- Hip and pelvis
- Spine (up)
- Spine (down)
- Spinal stimulation

Self-help

You will probably be at home for much of the first stage of labour when the cervix is dilating. Try the following to help you cope.

- Ask your partner to massage your lower back, working in small circles. Placing a hot-water bottle wrapped in a towel on the lower back may also help.

- Eat and drink little but often to build up your strength. Sip water and eat small amounts of carbohydrates such as toast, rice, pasta or bananas.

- Rest as much as possible to save your energy for what lies ahead.

Why not try?

Visualization – imagine that your baby is moving down and your cervix is opening like a flower to ease her passage. Think of a place or a colour that you find very soothing and focus on that instead of the pain.

Pituitary
Hold the right foot with your left hand. Starting at the base, creep up the big toe with your right thumb. Change hands to work the left foot.

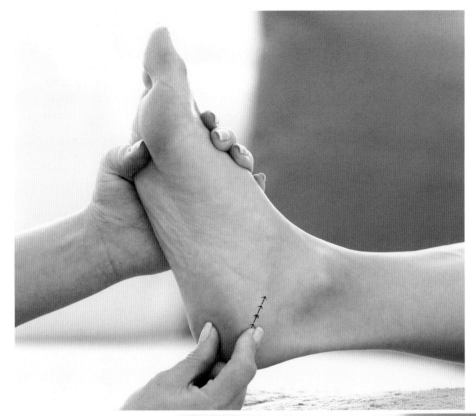

Uterus

Hold the right foot with your left hand. The reflex point for the uterus is between the heel and the ankle bone on the medial side, so work across this area from the tip of the heel with your right index finger. Change hands to work the left foot.

Coccyx

Hold the top of the right foot with your right hand. Creep up the inside of the heel area with the four fingers of your left hand. Change hands to treat the left foot.

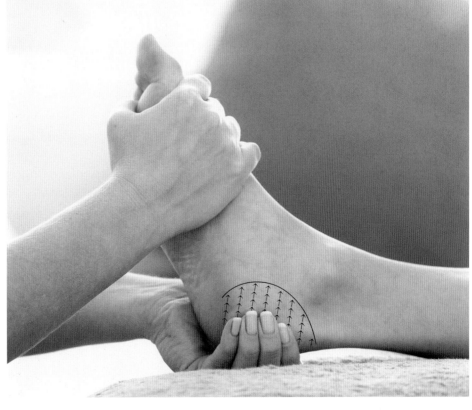

Hip and pelvis

Hold the right foot with your left hand. Using the fingers of your right hand, work the outside of the heel. Change hands to treat the left foot.

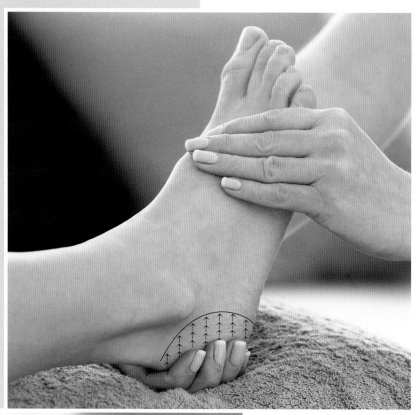

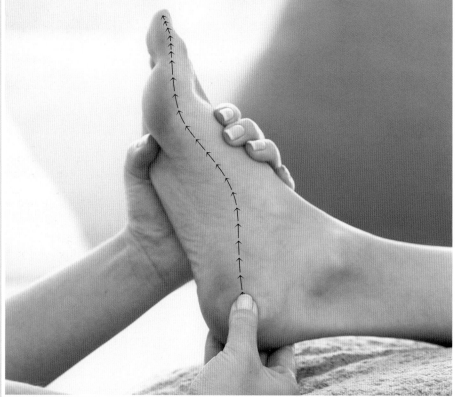

Spine (up)

Hold the right foot with your left hand. Using your right thumb, creep up the inside edge of the foot to the top of the big toe. Change hands to work the left foot.

Spine (down)

Use the back of your right hand to support the sole of the right foot. Use your left thumb to creep down the inside edge of the foot. Move your supporting hand down as you go. Change hands to treat the left foot.

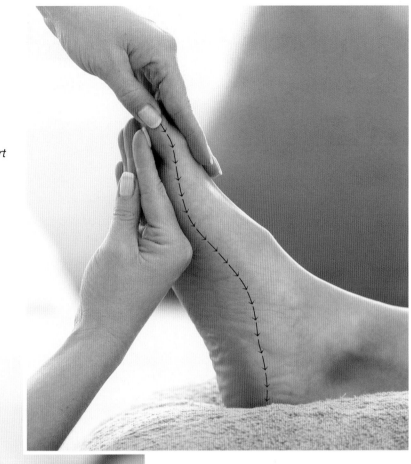

Spinal stimulation point

This reflex at the narrowest part of the foot on the medial side treats the whole of the central nervous system and the vertebral column. Hold the right foot with your left hand. Using your right thumb, press down on this point with a rotating movement towards the spine to a count of five. Pause and repeat. Change hands to work the left foot

Post-natal depression

You have reached the end of your pregnancy, gone through the experience of giving birth and you have held your precious baby in your arms – a wonderful, emotional feeling. You will marvel at the detail in every finger and toe, the tiny ears, perfect nose and mouth, and that soft downy skin.

You expected to feel on top of the world and some mothers do. Others though – and this is more common in first pregnancies – experience an overwhelming feeling of tension and anxiety, and are afraid they will be unable to cope. Many women suffer mild post-natal depression, known as 'baby blues' a few days after the birth, no matter how delighted they are with the new baby. They may become tearful, irritable and depressed, reactions mostly caused by the sudden hormonal changes in the body after the birth.

Also, the realization that this tiny person is totally dependent upon you for survival can be overwhelming at first. You may feel trapped and unable to fulfil the constant demands of the newborn.

Tiredness, too, can increase your feelings of depression and anxiety. Forty years ago it was usual for women to stay in hospital for ten days after a completely normal birth. If there were complications their stay was extended. Babies stayed in their cots by their mother's beds during the day, but for the first five nights they were taken out after the 10 p.m. feed and slept in the nursery. Mothers could then catch up on sleep and regain some of their strength after the exertion of giving birth.

Today a mother may give birth in the morning and be discharged in the evening, or the following day. There may be no time to escape from the demands of a family and enjoy some rest and quiet.

Looking after yourself

Even if you have no appetite, make sure that you do eat something every few hours. It is essential that you keep your blood sugar in balance to help you through this difficult time and to keep up your milk supply. Herbs such as St John's Wort can be useful remedies for depression, but some doctors believe that you should not take even herbal remedies while you are breastfeeding as anything you take can pass to your baby through your milk. Always seek medical advice.

Don't try to do too much and don't feel you have to do everything. Ask for help with the household chores so you have time to rest. Take a break once in a while – perhaps a friend or relative could mind your baby

Calming colic

One source of anxiety and depression for new mothers is evening colic – your baby cries and cries, showing signs of considerable discomfort and nothing you do seems to help. Breastfeeding mothers can help calm baby's colic while stimulating their milk supply by drinking infusions of chamomile, cinnamon, cardamom or fennel. Traces of these herbs and spices, all of which are good for digestion, will be passed on via the breast milk and may help sooth the colic.

for an hour or two so you can go out for a walk or take a relaxing bath. Try to find an hour or so in the evening when the baby is settled and you and your partner can have some time together alone.

Benefits of reflexology

Reflexology can be a great help at this time, helping to relax you, balance your hormones and energizing your system. It can also ease discomfort in the vaginal and rectal areas, relieve engorged breasts and encourage your milk supply. If your husband, partner, or friend can give you a relaxing reflexology treatment you will soon notice a difference.

Bonding with your baby
Getting to know your new baby is very exciting, but most new mothers have some difficult moments in the first few weeks.

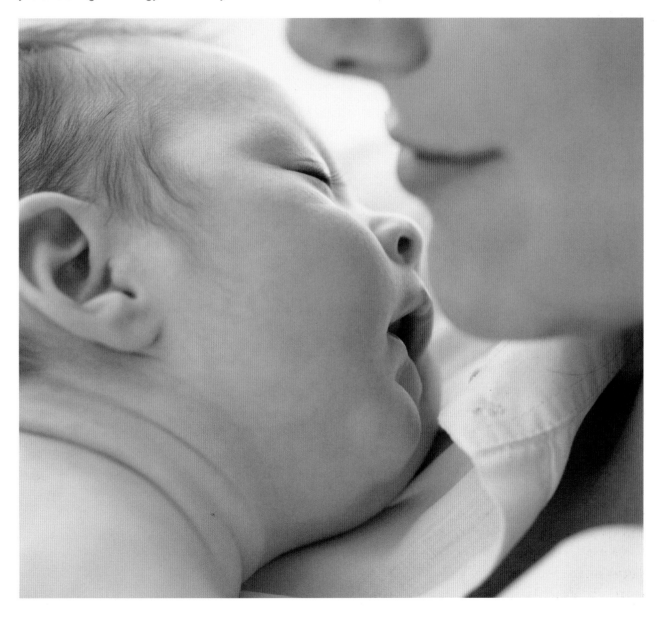

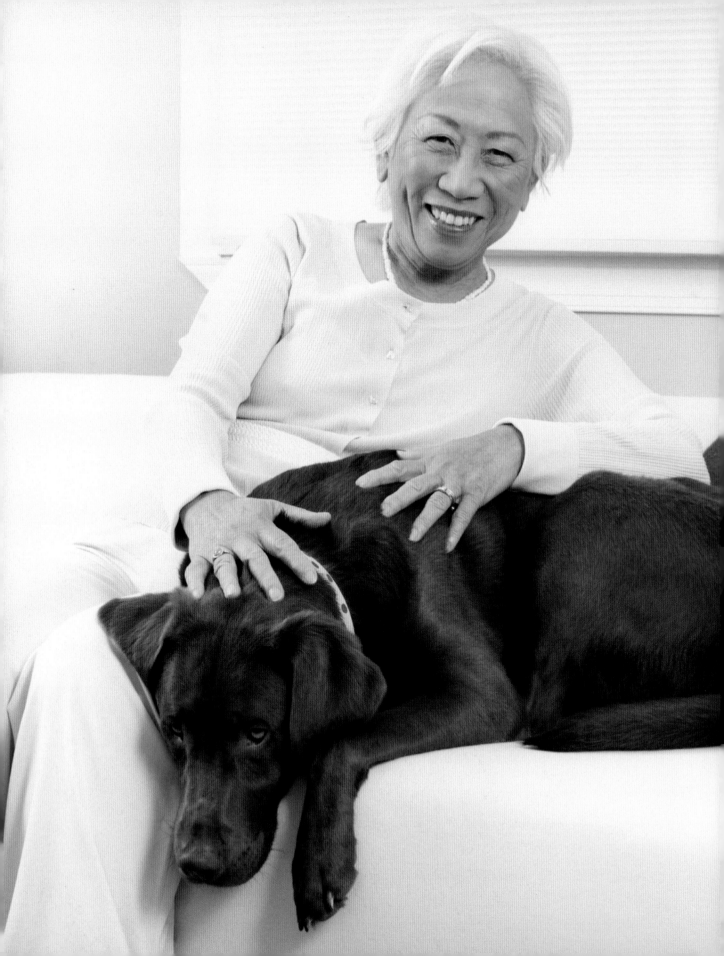

Reflexology in the later years

The human body has significant powers of self-healing and regeneration. In fact, the body likes being well and it fights a constant battle every day to defend us from harmful viruses and bacteria, sending out signals in the form of symptoms when things are going wrong.

If the body was not able to serve us so faithfully our joints and bones would be brittle by the age of 20, our arteries clogged with fatty deposits by the age of 35, and our brains would fail to retain any knowledge by the age of 45. There is a process of decay and regeneration going on every day of our lives so we can survive and stay healthy for longer. And today, given good living conditions, people in many countries are living longer than ever before.

But even in the developed nations malnutrition is all too common and many older people have a diet that is deficient in the vitamins and minerals necessary to help keep the body in a good state of repair. Just as we would not fail to have our car serviced regularly in order to prolong its life, we need to look after ourselves and keep a close check on our health. Reflexology can be of benefit in all manner of disorders, but for the best results it should be used as a general treatment to help keep the body healthy as well as when illness strikes.

A natural menopause

Just like the start of the menstrual cycle in your teens, the ending of your periods is a natural event, an indication that the childbearing years are over. I believe that there is no reason why the menopause should be regarded as an illness or something that needs medical intervention by way of drugs to help a woman through this period in her life. That said, many women do experience unpleasant symptoms such as hot flushes, night sweats, depression, insomnia, dry vagina, low libido and mood swings to varying degrees of severity.

Nature does provide for the time when the ovaries cease to produce oestrogen. Our adrenal glands make a form of oestrogen called oestrone

Self-help

Stress and poor eating habits all put strain on the adrenal system, so try making these simple dietary and lifestyle changes. They should reduce menopausal symptoms and make you feel better.

• Keep active and make sure you do regular exercise, such as walking, swimming or a light work-out in the gym.

• Reduce your intake of sugar and products containing white flour.

• Don't drink too much tea or coffee. One or two cups a day are enough, as tea and coffee can deplete the body of vital nutrients.

• Eat plenty of wholegrains, such as brown rice, wholemeal bread, oats, and wholemeal pasta.

• Increase your intake of essential fatty acids, particularly those sources rich in omega-3 fats, such as linseed, pumpkin seeds, oily fish, olive oil, tofu and green vegetables.

• Reduce your intake of dairy products. Rice milk or almond milk are both excellent substitutes for cow's milk and can be used on cereals and in cooking.

• If you are suffering from vaginal dryness, squeeze the oil from a vitamin E capsule into your vagina. You can also take a vitamin E supplement daily.

• Vitamin C is known for its beneficial effect on the immune system, but it is also an anti-inflammatory. It helps the body build up collagen, which is a protein and is the packing tissue between the organs in the body.

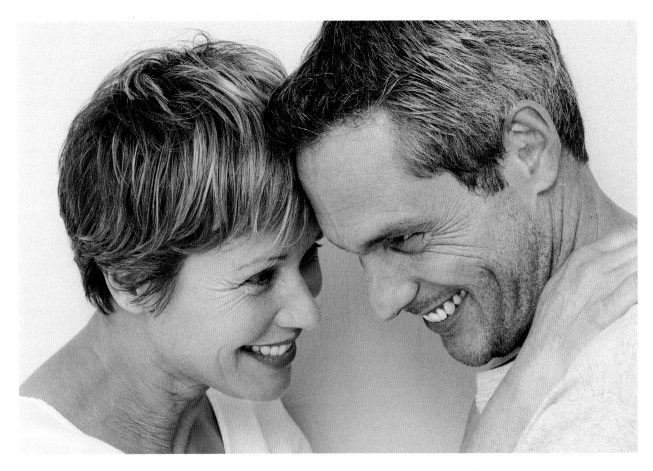

to provide the body with sufficient supplies of this hormone to help our bones and joints to remain strong, our hair and skin supple, and muscles toned. The stronger a woman's adrenal function, the easier her menopause will be.

A natural approach

If you go to your doctor with menopausal symptoms you may be offered hormone replacement therapy, which will certainly help your symptoms but is not without its own side-effects. Among these are an increased risk of breast/womb cancer, undesirable weight gain, bloating, depression and raised blood pressure. You may decide the advantages outweigh the disadvantages, but before embarking on hormone replacement therapy it is well worth trying some dietary and lifestyle changes and looking at a natural approach to the menopause. Reflexology can be of great help in reducing feelings of stress and tension during the menopause years and working on the hormonal system and adrenal glands can alleviate many of the distressing symptoms. If your adrenal reflex is very sensitive, you can be sure your adrenal glands have been overworking for too long.

Lift your mood
Depression can disrupt your life and your relationships. If you suffer from depression during the menopause, try taking St John's Wort. It can be as effective as antidepressants, which are sometimes prescribed for menopausal women.

Treating the menopause

The deeply relaxing effects of reflexology can really help reduce the feelings of stress and tension that are so common during the menopause. Most women find, too, that treatment on the endocrine system (pituitary and thyroid) helps control the hot flushes that are one of the most distressing symptoms. I also recommend working on the spinal area reflex to stimulate the nerve and blood supply to the whole body. Another way of treating symptoms is with herbs. Sage helps alleviate hot flushes, and black cohosh balances the hormonal system. These herbs are available in tablet form at healthfood shops and some chemists.

Areas to work

- Pituitary
- Thyroid (dorsal and plantar)
- Uterus
- Ovaries
- Spine
- Liver

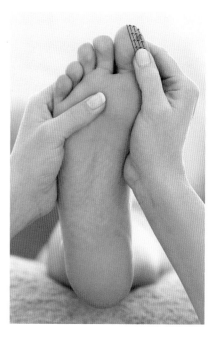

Pituitary
Hold the right foot with your left hand. Start by applying pressure to the base of the big toe, then creep up the big toe several times. Change hands to work the left foot.

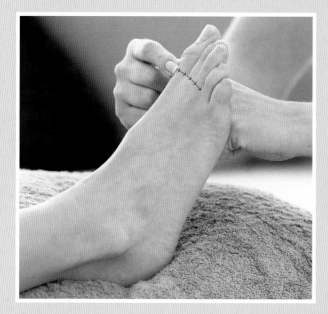

Thyroid (dorsal)
Support the right foot with your left fist. With your right index finger, creep along the bases of the first three toes. Change hands to work the left foot.

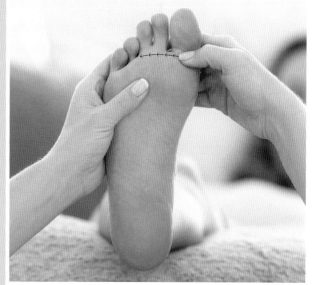

Thyroid (plantar)
Hold the right foot with your left hand. With your right thumb, creep along the base of the first three toes. Repeat three times. Change hands to treat the left foot.

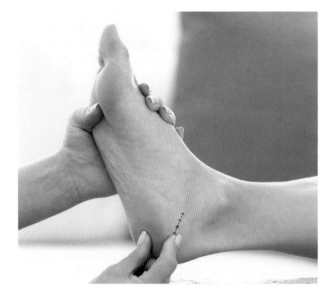

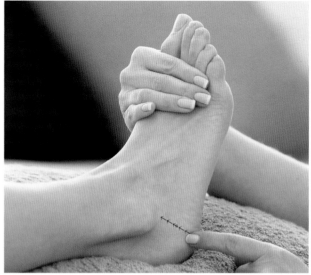

Uterus

Hold the right foot with your left hand. The reflex point for the uterus is between the heel and the ankle bone on the medial side, so work across this area from the tip of the heel with your right index finger. Change hands to work the left foot.

Ovaries

Hold the right foot with your right hand. The reflex point for the ovaries is between the heel and the ankle bone on the lateral side of the foot, so use your left index finger to creep from the tip of the heel to the ankle bone. Change hands to work the left foot.

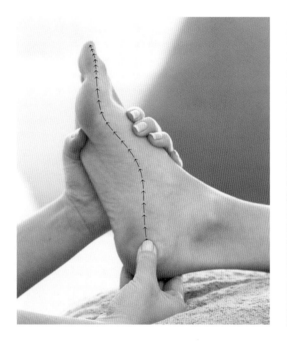

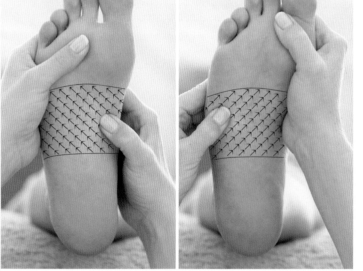

Spine

Hold the right foot with your left hand and with your right thumb, creep up the medial edge of the foot to the top of the big toe. Change hands to work the left foot.

Liver

The liver reflex is only on the right foot. Holding the foot with your left hand, creep across the reflex area with your right thumb. Work from the medial to the lateral side. Switch hands and work back in the opposite direction.

Back and bone conditions

As we get older, and perhaps less active, we lose muscle tone. This can cause pain in the lower back, hips, shoulders and knees. There is only one way of helping to keep our bones and joints as supple as possible and that is to keep moving.

We don't move around in our homes as we used to. We don't have to lay coal fires and sweep grates, polish floors and bash rugs on the clothes line – excellent exercise for the arms, shoulders and breasts as it encourages the lymph to move around the upper part of the body. Washing machines take the work out of washing clothes and even the television is operated by remote control so we don't have to move from our seat to change channels. Many of us spend hours in front of the computer and order the shopping online to be delivered to the door so we don't have to go to the supermarket. Our bodies become weaker, and back pain more common. It is so important to go for even just a short walk every day, have a swim in your local pool or enjoy a gentle work-out in the gym. If you keep moving, your muscles stay strong and they in turn will help prevent aches and pains.

Osteoporosis

Osteoporosis generally affects women (and sometimes men) over the age of 45–50. Among post-menopausal caucasian women osteoporosis is more common than heart attacks, strokes, diabetes, rheumatoid arthritis or breast cancer.

Healthy bones are dense and contain plenty of calcium and other minerals. Bones affected by osteoporosis lack minerals and become brittle and porous. In some people the bones get so fragile that they break and fracture very easily. The whole skeleton may be affected, but bone loss is usually worst in the spine, hips and ribs. Osteoporosis itself does not cause back pain, but it can result in pain if the vertebrae become so weak that they can no longer withstand normal stresses. Fragile bones lead to aches, pains and fractures in various parts of the body, especially the spine, neck, hips and shoulders. The sufferer is often unaware of the severity of the disease until she has a fall, perhaps fracturing a bone, and an X-ray reveals severe bone loss in many parts of the body.

There is no question that lowered oestrogen levels lead to bone loss. When a woman is going through the menopause the decline in oestrogen alters the secretion of hormones from other glands in the

body. Consequently the cells responsible for breaking down bone become a lot more active than those that build new bone.

Osteoporosis usually shows up 10 to 20 years after a natural menopause or within 4 to 11 years if a woman has had her ovaries removed before that time. Women who have an early menopause tend to be more prone to the disease, and on average women who smoke reach menopause five years earlier than non-smokers. Bone loss occurs 50 per cent faster among smokers. Drinking excessive amounts of coffee can also lead to increased bone loss because caffeine interferes with calcium absorption.

Other causes of osteoporosis

Further causes of osteoporosis include a malfunctioning adrenal, thyroid or parathyroid gland, too little vitamin D and an excessive use of diuretics and cortisone. Diuretics cause valuable minerals to be excreted from the bloodstream, especially potassium, and any drug that has a steroid/cortisone base depletes calcium from bone. Excessive alcohol also increases your risk of bone loss, and eating too much salt may leach calcium from the body.

Signs of osteoporosis

One simple indicator of osteoporosis is a decrease in height as bone mass declines. Another sign that may give warning of osteoporosis long before any spinal damage is tooth loss from peridontal disease. It is well known that gum inflammation is caused by the formation of plaque on the teeth. It is less well known that gum inflammation can also arise from bone degeneration. In animals that are deprived of calcium the jaw is the first bone to develop osteoporosis. When this happens the teeth loosen enough to irritate the gums and cause inflammation. Tooth loss in caucasian women between 60 and 70 has been strongly correlated with the loss of bone density elsewhere in the body.

Osteomalacia

Osteomalacia causes a weakness of bone but the bones usually soften, unlike osteoporosis when the bones become thin and brittle. The main cause of osteomalacia is a deficiency of vitamin D caused by a poor diet, lack of sunshine or both. The deficiency leads to progressive decalcification of bony tissues, causing bone pain. Pains in the long bones of the arms and legs are common, as well as pain in the vertebral column. Sufferers must take vitamin D supplements.

Exercise

Exercise is essential, but there has to be a good balance; too much can cause stress on thin bones. Walking is the one of the simplest and best ways to exercise – 30 minutes a day is recommended – combined with lots of stretching exercises. Bone growth requires the expending of effort against the resistance of gravity. If you are very active, therefore, skipping is a great form of exercise.

Rheumatism

Rheumatism is any disorder in which aches and pains affect the muscles and joints. This means that rheumatic pains can come and go and rarely cause any long-term serious disability.

Rheumatism is derived from the Greek word *rheuma*, meaning a flow, which describes a watery discharge within the joints that frequently accompanies the inflammation and pain in joints and muscles. Some people experience rheumatic pain when the weather changes and becomes cold and damp.

Arthritis

Arthritis is a very different form of disease. The name comes from the Greek word *arthron*, meaning joint, and *itis*, meaning inflammation. The word arthritis, therefore, means an inflamed joint. In osteoarthritis, the most common form, the normally smooth cartilage in a healthy joint becomes rough and flaky. The joint is less resilient and more easily strained and damaged, causing pain and stiffness. Over the age of 45 osteoarthritis is ten times more common in women than men. Weight-bearing joints, particularly hips, knees and spines, are worst affected so it is important to avoid becoming overweight, which puts yet more strain on joints.

Eat your greens
Arthritis sufferers need a balanced diet that provides important vitamins and minerals and keeps weight down. Meals should include plenty of fresh, nutrient-packed vegetables.

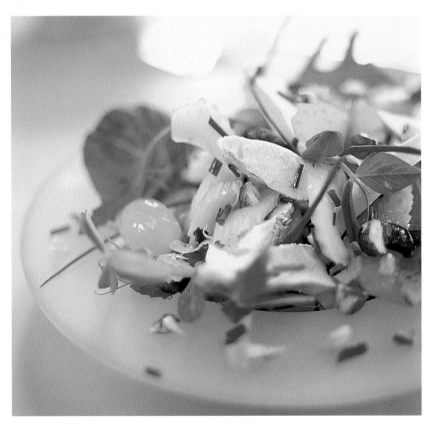

Causes of arthritis

Researchers are still unable to explain what causes the disease in the first place. One theory is that arthritis results from some sort of infection, yet no infectious agent has been singled out. Stress, while it does not actually cause arthritis, appears to have a major role to play since stress can weaken the resistance of the body in general. Many people are diagnosed with arthritis after a very emotionally stressful episode in their lives. Excessive stresses and strains or regular exposure to cold and dampness can similarly lead to local weaknesses of the bones and joints. Some scientists believe that mineral and vitamin deficiencies may play a part in succumbing to the disease in the first place.

It is worth trying herbs that have an anti-inflammatory action for relieve from pain of arthritis. These include feverfew, circumin, Korean ginseng and devil's claw. It also helps to cut sugar out of your diet, and that includes all the hidden sugars in cakes, biscuits and pastries. Sugar causes the blood to become very acidic, which makes the condition worse. Use only the minimum of salt too and try enhancing the flavour in your foods by using herbs instead. Omega-3 supplements are very beneficial for inflammatory conditions.

Self-help

Keep your bones healthy by eating sensibly and taking vitamin and mineral supplements if necessary.

• After the age of 35 a woman needs at least 1200 milligrams of calcium daily to prevent bone loss. Eat calcium-rich foods such as milk and dairy products and dark green leafy vegetables, and take a supplement if necessary.

• The body needs vitamin D for calcium to be absorbed. Vitamin D is made by the body when the skin is exposed to sunlight, so short exposure to sunshine whenever possible is recommended.

• About 45 per cent of living bone consists of minerals, primarily calcium, phosphorus and magnesium. Calcium and phosphorus are required in equal amounts. The reason you seldom hear much said about the benefits of phosphorus for healthy bones is because many of us get too much phosphorus from artificial foods such as fizzy drinks and excess phosphorus can upset the calcium balance in the body. The right way to include phosphorus in your daily diet is to eat wholegrains and all forms of beans, and green vegetables.

• Make sure you have at least 100 milligrams of vitamin C a day, preferably from foods such as citrus fruit and broccoli. Vitamin C aids the formation of cartilage, which is a dense connective tissue produced by the body to cover the surface of bones, particularly at joints, where wear and damage occurs the most.

Rheumatoid arthritis

This is a rather different form of arthritis and although it still affects the joints and bones the cause is quite complex. Rheumatoid arthritis tends to occur in the 30–50 age group and is more common in women than men and in people over the age of 40. Normally your immune system helps to protect you against infections, but in rheumatoid arthritis it attacks the joints, particularly the lining of joints, instead, causing swelling and pain. The hands and feet are usually affected first, but the condition can spread to any synovial joint.

There is no cure at present, but a healthy diet with plenty of fruit, vegetables and wholegrain foods, and reduced meat, sugar, refined carbohydrate and saturated fats does seem to help many sufferers. Some people find it helpful to avoid certain foods, such as red meats and plants of the deadly nightshade family (tomato, potato, aubergine and peppers). Oily fish is beneficial as it helps reduce inflammation. Cod liver oil is also helpful. Take one tablespoon mixed with two tablespoons of fresh milk first thing every morning.

Treating bone conditions

Reflexology can be of great benefit in treating all the conditions relating to the skeletal system described on pages 94–97 and easing the aches and pains common in our more mature years. It can bring relief from pain, more mobility in joints and a better quality of life.

I recommend treating the digestive system as well as working on the spine and limbs. This increases the body's efficiency at absorbing the necessary vitamins and minerals and also helps to eliminate toxins as efficiently as possible.

Areas to work

- Coccyx
- Hip and pelvis
- Chronic neck
- Shoulder (dorsal and plantar)
- Spine
- Knee and elbow
- Liver
- Stomach and pancreas
- Intestines
- Illeocecal valve
- Sigmoid colon and rectum

Coccyx
Supporting the top of the right foot with your right hand, creep up the medial side of the heel with the four fingers of your left hand. Change hands to work the left foot.

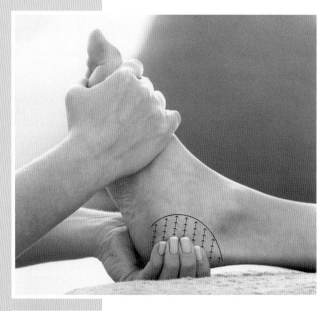

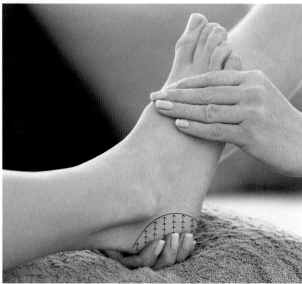

Hip and pelvis
Supporting the top of the right foot with your right hand, creep up the lateral side of the heel with the four fingers of your left hand. Change hands to work the left foot.

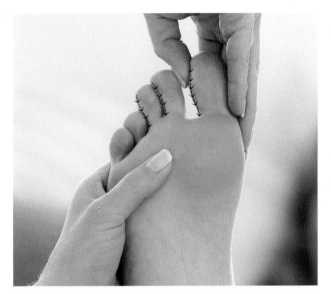

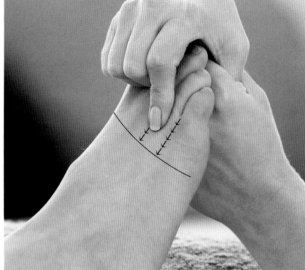

Chronic neck

This treatment helps all chronic neck conditions, especially in older people. Hold the right foot with your left hand. Work down the lateral sides of the first three toes with your right thumb, starting with the big toe. Change hands to work the left foot.

Shoulder (dorsal)

Push your left fist against the sole of the right foot. Work down the grooves of the fourth and fifth toes with your right index finger. Change hands to work the left foot.

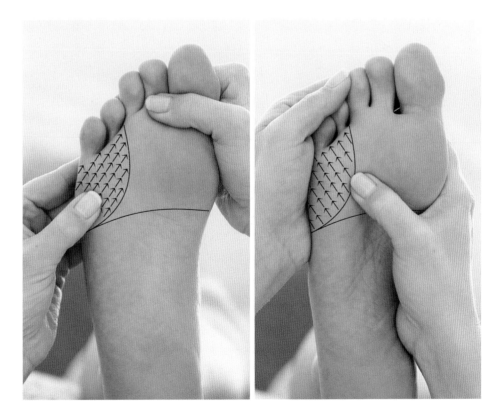

Shoulder (plantar)

Cradle the top of the right foot with your right hand. Use your left thumb to creep across the shoulder reflex area. Then change hands and creep back again across the area with your right thumb. Change hands to work the left foot.

Spine

Hold the right foot with your left hand. Creep up the inside edge of the foot to the top of the big toe with your right thumb. Change hands to work the left foot.

The spinal column is the most important reflex area to work on because nerves arising from the spine stimulate the entire body and improve nerve and blood supply, helping to detoxify and encourage the healing process.

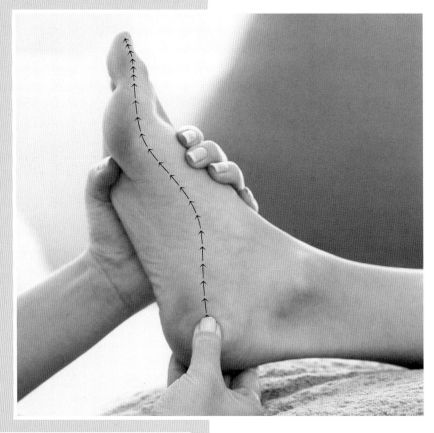

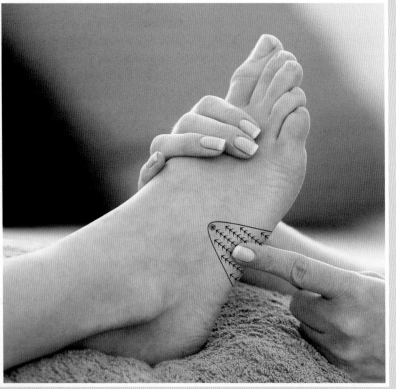

Knee and elbow

Hold the right foot with your left hand. Creep your right index finger up the triangular-shaped reflex on the lateral side of the foot. Change hands to work the left foot.

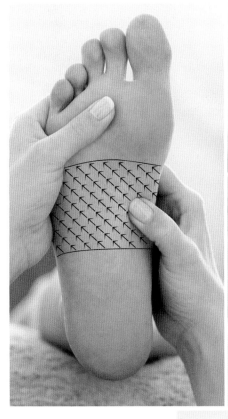

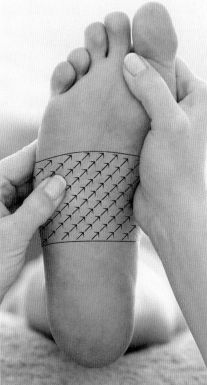

Liver
This is a good area to work on for hormonal problems as the liver gets rid of excess hormones. The liver reflex is on the right foot only. Hold the foot with your left hand. Creep your right thumb across, at the angle shown (far left), working from the medial to the lateral side. Change hands and work back with your left thumb (left).

Stomach and pancreas
The main reflex for the stomach area is on the left foot only, between the diaphragm line and the waist line (see page 10). Support the foot with your right hand. Work over the area shown with your left thumb, moving from the medial to the lateral side of the foot (right). Change hands and work back across the area with your right thumb (far right).

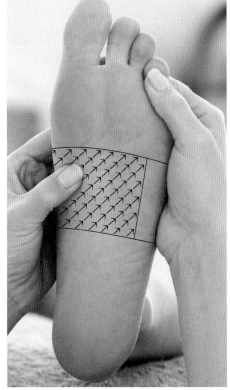

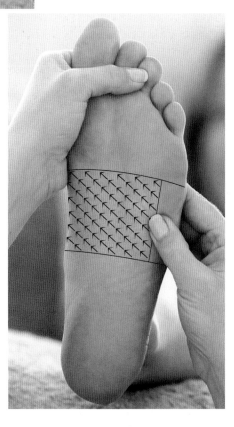

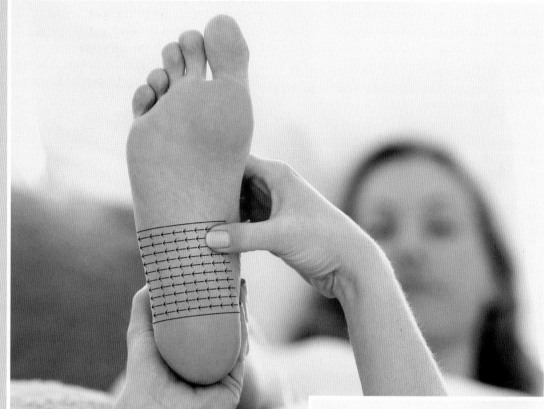

Intestines

Supporting the right foot with your left hand, work over the area below the waist line (see page 10) with your right thumb. Work in straight lines from the medial to the lateral side of the foot.

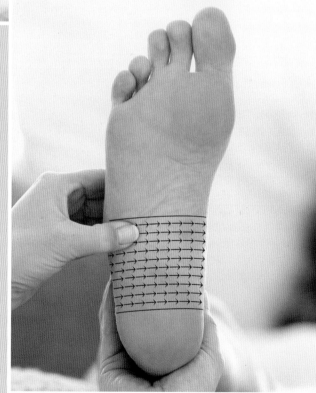

Intestines

Change hands and work back across the area with your left thumb. Work in straight lines as before, but from the lateral to the medial side. Change hands to work the left foot.

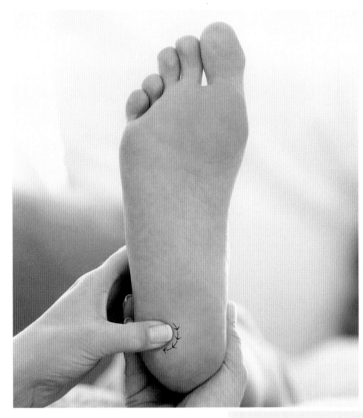

Ileocecal valve
This reflex is only on the right foot. Hold the foot with your right hand. Find the reflex, which lies below the pelvic line (see page 10) on the lateral side of the foot, and work with the left thumb, using the hooking-out technique (see page 13).

Sigmoid colon and rectum
Found only on the left foot, this V-shaped reflex area lies under the pelvic line (see page 10). Holding the foot with your left hand, work up the inside fork of the reflex area with your right thumb (right). Change hands and work up the outside fork with your left thumb.

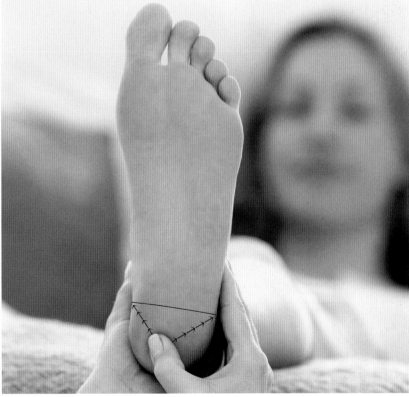

Heart and lungs

Heart disease is still a leading causes of death in the Western world and many women as well as men suffer from heart attacks and angina pain. Common causes of heart problems include too much stress, lack of exercise, emotional conflicts, smoking, and a diet rich in salt, sugar and fat. Too much fat is particularly damaging to the heart and can cause fatty deposits to build up in the walls of the arteries. If you smoke you must stop altogether for a heart condition to improve.

The heart is a tough muscle, about the size of its owner's fist. It starts beating on the 16th day after conception and can continue for a hundred years or more without breaking down, needing replacement parts or even a service! No machine pump could ever be so efficient.

If anything goes wrong with the heart there is an adverse effect on the whole body, which is manifested through one or more distressing symptoms, such as palpitations, breathlessness, fatigue, chest pain or blackouts. Reflexology can help treat heart disease by reducing stress levels, improving nerve and muscle function and increasing the blood supply to the heart.

Angina

Angina is a pain or uncomfortable strangulated feeling in the chest brought on by too little oxygen reaching the heart muscle. The heart is crying out for more oxygen-rich blood which is being deprived from it

Self-help

A balanced diet is vital for a healthy heart. The heart needs the correct amounts of proteins, carbohydrates, fats and minerals such as potassium, sodium, magnesium and calcium.

• Cut down on fat and salt, eat plenty of fruit and vegetables (at least five portions a day) and try to stay a healthy weight.

• Regular physical exercise is essential and so is mental relaxation. Try meditation, letting your thoughts wander as you listen to relaxing music, massage, reflexology, tai chi, or yoga.

• Angry, hostile emotions can raise blood pressure and consequently affect the heart. When you are under stress, there is a rise in pulse rate, an increase in oxygen demand by the tissues and an increase in cardiac output.

Self-help

To keep your respiratory system healthy and avoid bronchitis, try the following tips.

• Avoid mucus-making foods like dairy products. Milk and cheese in particular can clog the bronchial tubes.

• Eat plenty of onions and garlic and lots of citrus fruits, such as lemons, oranges and grapefruit to boost your vitamin C intake. Make a soothing drink of freshly squeezed lemon juice, hot water and a spoonful of honey.

• Avoid using chemical sprays in your home, such as oven cleaners, carpet cleaners or room perfumes, as the fumes from these sprays can affect your lungs.

• Practise deep breathing to expand your lung capacity. Take a deep breath in through your mouth, directing the breath to your navel area. Breathe out slowly, contracting the abdominal muscles to exhale as much air as you can. Repeat.

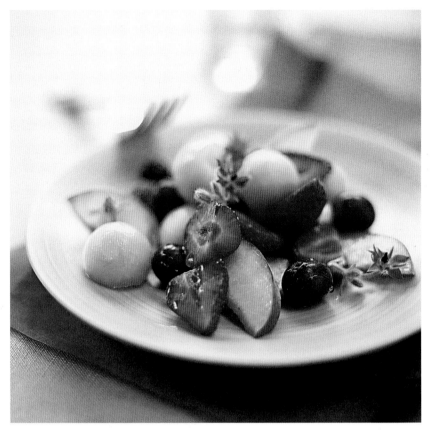

A healthy plateful
Packed with vitamins, all kinds of berries are good for the heart and the blood. Try to eat some every day.

due to congestion in the arteries. Angina pain usually comes on with exertion or anxiety and is relieved by resting for a while. Pain generally starts in the centre of the chest, behind the breastbone and sometimes travels to the arms, usually the left arm, and can even affect the fingers. After the menopause, angina is as common in woman as in men. Angina is generally caused by coronary artery disease or a narrowing of the artery caused by fatty deposits in the artery walls. High blood pressure, high blood cholesterol and smoking all increase the risk of angina.

Bronchitis

Bronchitis can affect people of any age, but the very young and very old are particularly vulnerable, especially in winter. Smokers are also particularly likely to suffer bronchitis. Symptoms are coughing, wheezing and breathlessness, caused by sticky mucus deposits in the airways. The bronchial tubes become obstructed and inflamed and breathing is difficult. Doctors can prescribe antibiotics to reduce the infection and maybe an inhaler to open up the airways to allow a better flow of oxygen to the lungs. Reflexology treatment can ease the symptoms of bronchitis and help build up resistance to the condition.

Dos and don'ts

• DO exercise at least four times a week.

• DO walk or cycle short distances instead of driving.

• DO take the stairs instead of the lift. Walk up escalators.

• DO eat regular meals, with salads and fresh vegetables every day.

• DO learn a form of relaxation such as meditation and practise it every day.

• DON'T smoke – every cigarette is another nail in your coffin.

• DON'T drink too much – one or two units of alcohol a day is more than enough.

• DON'T eat too much sugar or too many fried foods.

• DON'T let angry, stressful thoughts fester in your mind. Talk them through, resolve them and forget about them.

Treating heart and lung conditions

Both heart and chest conditions respond well to reflexology. Treatment helps muscular function, improves blood supply and nerve functioning, and boosts general health by reducing stress levels. Long-term reflexology can also lower blood pressure. The heart is associated with the left-hand side of the body and you will find the reflex points mostly on the left foot.

Reflexology is also successful in treating chest conditions such as emphysema, asthma and bronchitis.

Areas to work

- Heart
- Lung (plantar and dorsal)
- Ribcage relax

Keep blood pressure down

High blood pressure or hypertension is a common problem in older people. Here are some tips for keeping it down.

- Cut out or reduce your intake of alcohol and caffeine. Eat more fibre and less salt.

- Try not to get stressed. If you do, practise deep breathing.

- Take regular exercise, but check with your doctor before starting anything new.

Heart

The main heart reflex lies above the diaphragm line and beneath the first three toes. It is only on the left foot. Hold the foot with your right hand and creep across the area below the big toe to the third toe with your left thumb. Don't treat this reflex more than three times as you will also work it when treating the lung. The two reflexes overlap just as the organs do.

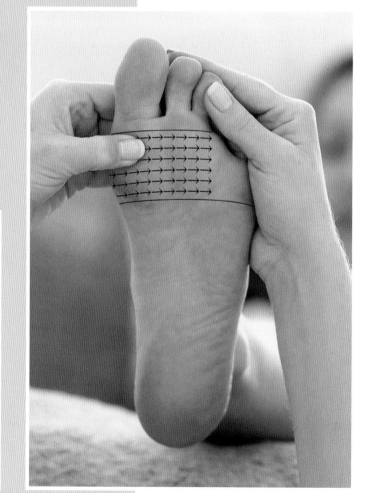

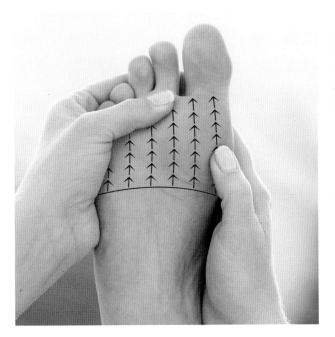

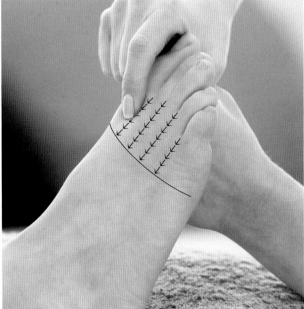

Lung (plantar)

Holding the right foot with your left hand, creep up the areas between the grooves of each toe on the sole of the foot with your right thumb. Change hands to work the left foot.

Lung (dorsal)

Press your left fist into the sole of the right foot. Creep down the grooves below the toes on the top of the foot with your right index finger. Change hands to work the left foot.

Ribcage relax

Press both your thumbs into the sole of the foot while creeping across the top of the foot with the fingers of both hands.

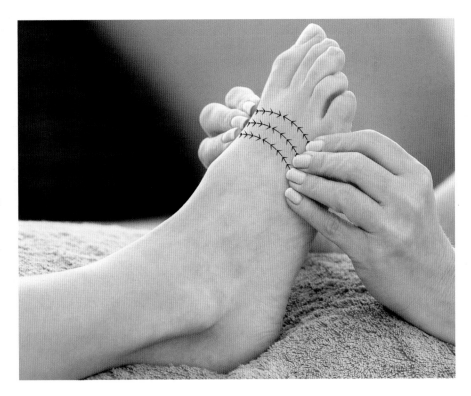

Problems for the elderly

These days many people continue living healthy active lives in their seventies, eighties and even nineties. But as you grow older, you are more likely to suffer some physical discomforts.

Incontinence

Many women have stress incontinence – leaking small amounts of urine when coughing, laughing, sneezing or lifting something heavy. The problem often starts after childbirth, particularly after a forceps delivery, which can weaken the muscles of the pelvic floor so they don't tighten properly. The pelvic floor muscles help keep the bladder outlet closed, but if they are weak, they cannot cope with extra stress or pressure and small amounts of urine may leak. A similar slackening in the muscles can come with age and many older women suffer from stress incontinence.

Pelvic floor exercises to strengthen pelvic floor muscles (see box) solve the problem for many people. If you have trouble with the exercises, see your doctor who can refer you to a special nurse or a physiotherapist for advice. Frequent reflexology treatments after childbirth can help prevent stress incontinence. Reflexology can also help reduce the severity if you are already suffering from incontinence. There are surgical procedures if all else fails.

Alzheimer's disease and dementia

Dementia is a term used to describe a condition that affects some older people, causing symptoms such as memory loss, confusion and poor concentration. Alzheimer's disease is the most common form of dementia, affecting one in ten people over the age of 65, and one in five of those over 80. The disease causes changes in the structure and chemistry of the brain, leading to the death of brain cells. The sufferer eventually loses all memory, and the personality changes and slowly disintegrates. He or she may

Pelvic floor exercises

To find out where your pelvic floor muscles are, imagine you are trying to stop the flow of urine and avoid passing wind at the same time. You will feel the muscles around your vagina and back passage tighten. Try not to pull in your tummy, tighten your buttock muscles or squeeze your legs together.

Hold your pelvic floor muscles as tightly as you can for as long as you can, building up to ten seconds. Repeat up to ten times, resting for four seconds between each squeeze.

Once you are used to the action, try doing the exercise quickly. Pull in your pelvic floor and hold for one second, then release. Repeat up to ten times.

Try to do a set of slow contractions and a set of quick contractions five or six times a day. You can do the exercises when sitting or lying down, but it's probably best to do them while standing up. If your symptoms don't improve after a couple of months, see your doctor.

become aggressive and destructive, which is heart-breaking for relatives and friends to watch.

Causes of Alzheimer's

There is often a shortage of certain chemicals in the brain of an Alzheimer's patient, but no one yet knows exactly what triggers the illness. There may be a number of factors involved, including age, genetic and environmental considerations, diet and general health. It is likely that in most cases a combination of these factors is responsible. Smokers and people who have high blood pressure or high cholesterol have an increased risk of Alzheimer's, as well as those who have suffered severe head injuries in the past.

The theory that Alzheimer's might be linked to exposure to aluminium in cooking pans is now generally thought to be unlikely. Links to mercury in dental amalgam have also been suggested, but there is no evidence for this. High alcohol intake causes the body to become dehydrated and dehydration affects brain cells. I recommend that we should all drink more water and keep our alcohol intake to a minimum, particularly in our later years.

There is no cure as yet for Alzheimer's, only treatment to reduce symptoms, such as tranquillisers. Reflexology treatment can be of benefit, reducing stiffness as well as mental symptoms such as restlessness and anxiety. I recommend treating the spine and brain reflexes, daily if at all possible. Other complementary therapies, such as aromatherapy and massage, may also help and many patients seem to find the personal contact and physical touch cheering. There is also some evidence that taking ginkgo biloba brings some improvement in mental functioning and behaviour and more research is underway.

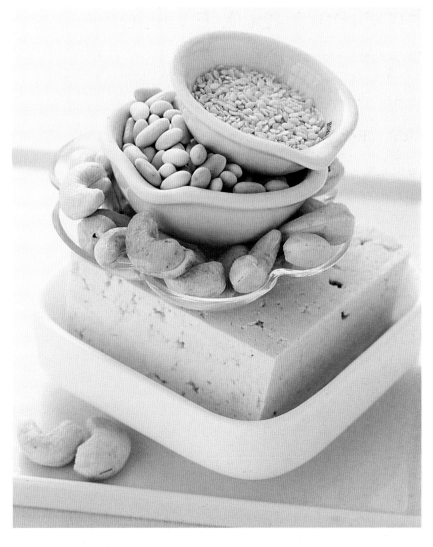

Zinc-rich foods
Zinc helps keep the brain healthy so eat foods rich in zinc such as oysters, beans, nuts, cheese and wholegrains or take a supplement. Vitamin B6 helps the body to absorb this mineral.

Treating the elderly

Reflexology can be of great benefit to the elderly, helping to ease general aches and pain as well as encouraging a feeling of well-being. For serious conditions, such as dementia, it is an ideal complementary therapy, but always make sure the patient's doctors are aware of the treatment and of any herbal remedies being taken.

Areas to work for incontinence
• Urinary system

Areas to work for dementia
• Head and neck
• Chronic neck
• Spine
• Brain

Why not try?

The herbs ladies' mantle and horsetail – both can be helpful for treating stress incontinence and strengthen muscle tone.

Urinary system
Hold the top of the right foot with your left hand. Using your right thumb, creep up the inside edge of the pelvic line (see page 10). Continue as far as the waist line (see page 10). Use the rotating technique (see page 13) to work the kidney reflex, just above where the waist and ligament lines cross. Change hands to work the left foot.

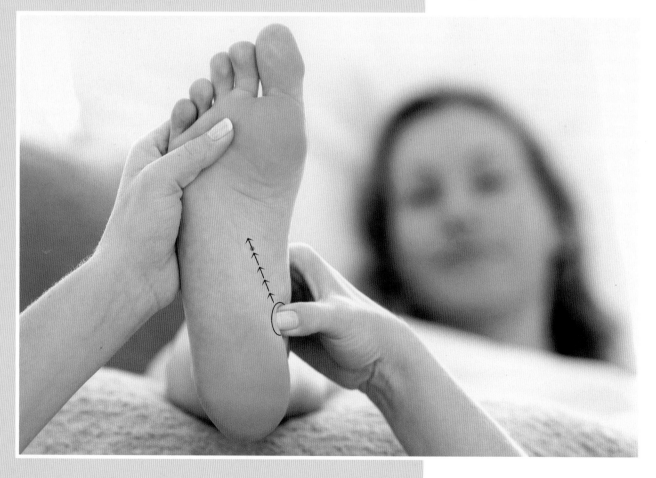

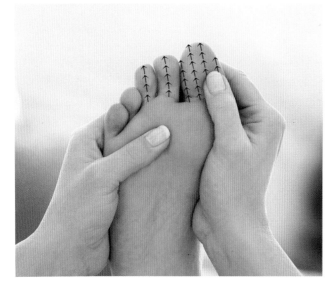

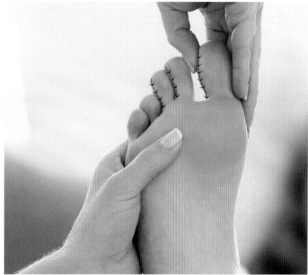

Head and neck

This treats all areas from the back of the neck to the top of the head. Hold the right foot with your left hand and use your right thumb to apply pressure and creep up the underside of the big, second and third toes. Change hands to work the left foot.

Chronic neck

This treatment is helpful for all chronic neck conditions, especially in older people. Hold the right foot with your left hand. Work down the sides of the first three toes with your right thumb as shown above, starting with the big toe. Change hands to work the left foot.

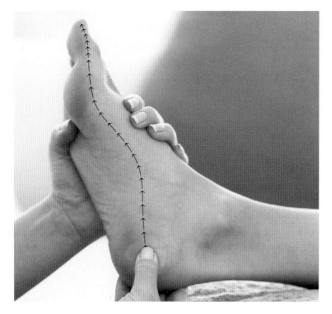

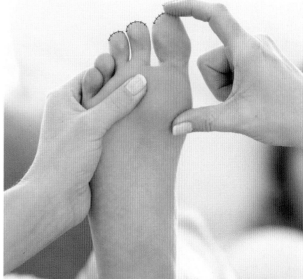

Spine

Hold the right foot with your left hand. Creep up the inside edge of the foot with your right thumb, then change to your index finger and creep up the big toe. The spine is the most important reflex area to work on because nerves arising from the spine stimulate the entire body.

Brain

After treating the spine, continue to work from the big toe over the top of the first three toes with your right index finger to make contact with the brain area. Change hands to work the left foot, starting with the spine area (see left) and continuing over the brain area.

Breast cancer

Breast cancer is one of the most common of all cancers in women. It can happen at any age, but the majority of sufferers are over 50. Fortunately, breast cancer is also one of the most treatable cancers and the rate of successful treatment and survival is encouragingly high. However, in my view, not enough research is being done on ways to prevent the disease from occurring in the first place.

We do know that a high-fibre diet decreases the risk whereas a high fat diet increases it. If you eat plenty of high-fibre food, the bowels, which are the body's waste disposal unit, are able to absorb more of the toxins that would otherwise find their way into the bloodstream. The advice is to cut down on animal fats, especially dairy foods such as cheese and butter, and eat plenty of fruit, vegetables and wholegrain foods. Tomatoes contain a carotenoid called lycopene which has anti-cancer properties, so eat some every day.

Research also shows that eating plenty of soya-rich foods may reduce the risk of breast cancer. In Japan and China where women consume high levels of soya there is a low incidence of breast cancer. The breast tissue of women with a soya-rich diet is less dense than that of women with low-soya diets and higher density breast tissue has shown to be linked to higher incidence of breast cancer. Soya contains plant oestrogens and these may interact with the female hormone oestrogen to lower levels of oestrogen in the body. High oestrogen levels seem to increase risk of breast cancer.

Risk factors

The established risk factors for breast cancer are age, oestrogen exposure (early onset of periods, late menopause, delayed pregnancy) as well as a family history of breast cancer. But I believe there may be other factors, too. With microwave ovens and many other electronic devices in the home that throw off radiation when they are in use, we have more radiation exposure in our daily lives now than ever before, and in my opinion this may be another cause of cancer.

Underarm antiperspirants 'seal in' perspiration, stopping the body being able to perspire naturally and throw out harmful toxins from the lymphatic glands under the arms. It is far better to use just a deodorant most of the time – it won't stop perspiration but will prevent odour – and save the antiperspirant for occasional use. Some say there is no risk from antiperspirants, but I believe it is best to avoid them if possible.

Lower your risk

The following are all believed to lower your risk of breast cancer.

• Avoiding excess weight.

• Eating a healthy diet with plenty of fruit and vegetables and wholegrains.

• Taking regular exercise.

• Not smoking.

• Avoiding too much alcohol.

• Research has also shown that women who have had a first child before the age of 30 and have breastfed are at lower risk of breast cancer.

Any form of stress, be it emotional or physical, reduces the efficiency of our immune system so increases the risk of cancer. And there are now warnings that the contraceptive pill, which alters the delicate function of the hormonal system, may have links with breast and other cancers.

If you do have breast cancer, or any other form of cancer, I do recommend having regular reflexology to aid your immune system and help the body heal itself. It is perfectly acceptable to receive reflexology alongside your medical treatment, but do always tell your doctors.

Keep fit and lower your risk
Taking plenty of physical exercise has been proven to reduce the risk of breast and uterine cancer. If you do have cancer, exercise also improves your chance of recovery.

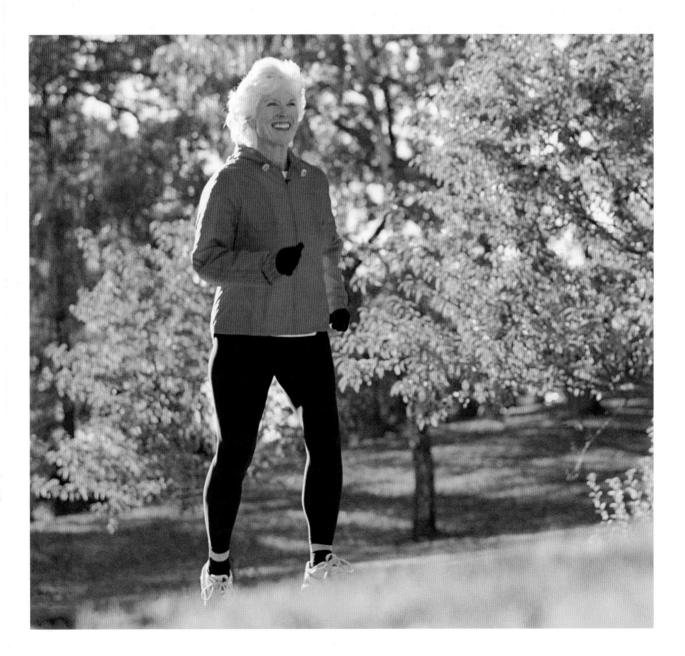

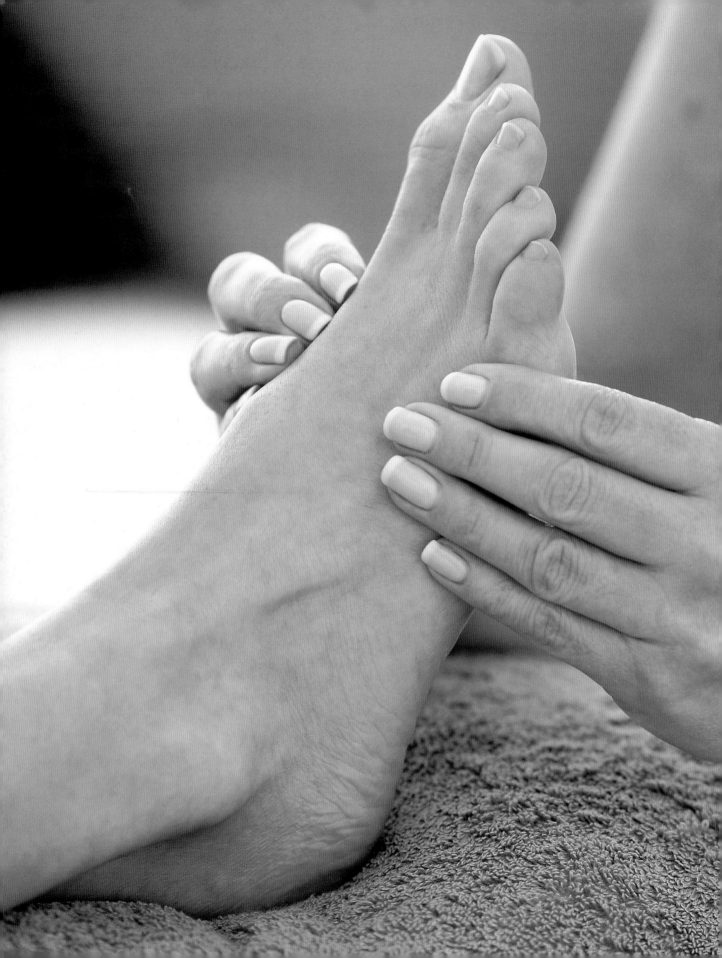

A complete
reflexology session

Easy to use and deeply relaxing, reflexology works to
restore your body's power to heal itself. It is not difficult
to follow the instructions in this book and conduct a
reflexology session on your friends or partner. Start
by giving a full treatment for the whole body before
moving on to work on particular areas as suggested
in the previous chapters. Both feet must be treated and
I recommend that you start with the right foot and then
go on to the left. Try to find a quiet, comfortable area
in your home where you can give or receive treatment
undisturbed. Some people like to talk during treatment.
Others prefer peace and quiet. You might like to play
some soothing music, or light a perfumed candle to
enhance the restful atmosphere.

A complete treatment is best, but if you only have
15 minutes or so to spare and your friend or partner
has severe period pains or is suffering from a headache
or back pain, try working on the coccyx, hip and pelvis,
and spinal areas. This is a general first aid-treatment
that will bring some relief.

A word of caution – ask a doctor or a professional
reflexologist for advice before treating anyone with a
serious illness, such as a heart condition or cancer.

Complete foot treatment

A complete reflexology treatment takes about 45 minutes. Ask the person receiving the treatment to lie down or sit on a comfortable chair with her feet on a pillow. The person giving the treatment should sit on a low stool with the receiver's feet on her lap.

The warm-up

Cover the receiver's legs and feet with a towel and apply a little talcum powder or light moisturizer to the feet. Start with the foot relaxation exercises (1–9) to ease any tension in the receiver and help make the feet feel supple and flexible.

The full routine

Treat both feet, whichever side of the body is suffering from pain or illness. Complete the sequence on the right foot first and then treat the left foot. As a general rule work on each reflex area twice, and if any reflex appears to be more sensitive, work over that area again. Always end the session with some of the relaxation treatments you gave at the beginning.

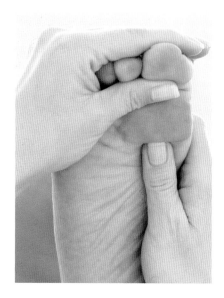

1 Diaphragm relax
Hold the right foot with your left hand. Press your right thumb into the start of the diaphragm line and work across to the lateral side, bending the toes over your left thumb. Change hands to treat the left foot.

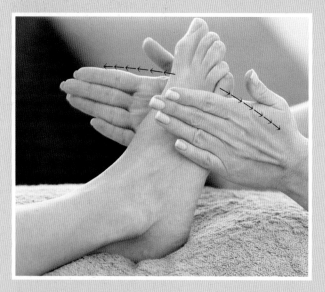

2 Side-to-side relax
Hold the foot between your hands and rock it from side to side between your palms. Your movements should be rapid but gentle. Repeat with the other foot.

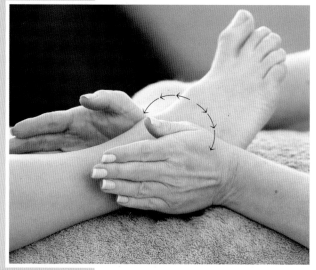

3 Ankle freeing
Hold the foot with the fleshy parts of your thumbs supporting the ankle bones. Keeping your wrists loose and relaxed, rock the foot from side to side gently but rapidly. Don't force the foot. This is a very good treatment for arthritis sufferers.

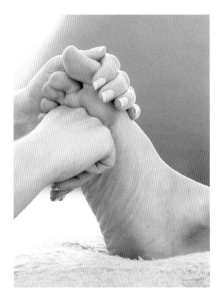

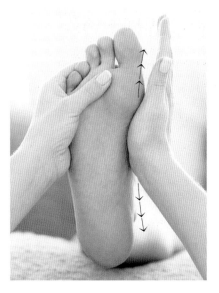

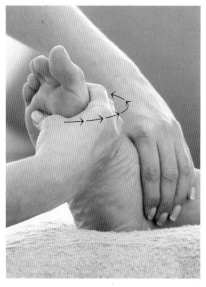

4 Metatarsal kneading

Push your right fist into the sole of the right foot. Squeeze the top of the foot with your left hand as if you are kneading dough. Change hands to treat the left foot.

5 Spinal friction

Hold the right foot with your left hand. With the flat of your right hand rub up and down the medial edge to stimulate the spinal column. Change hands to treat the left foot.

6 Circling: overgrip

Hold the right ankle with your left hand, your thumb on the lateral edge of the foot. Using your right hand, circle the foot towards the spine. Change hands for the left foot.

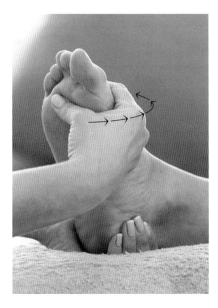

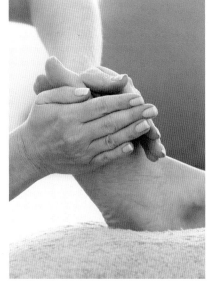

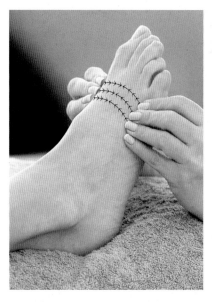

7 Circling: undergrip

Hold the heel of the right foot with your left hand. Using your right hand, gently circle the foot inwards and towards the spine. Change hands for the left foot.

8 Foot moulding

Hold the top of the right foot between your palms, then gently rotate your hands around the foot with movements like the motion of a steam train. Repeat with the left foot.

9 Ribcage relax

Press both your thumbs into the sole of the foot while creeping across the top of the foot with the fingers of both hands. Repeat with the left foot.

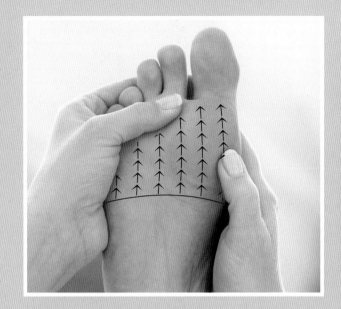

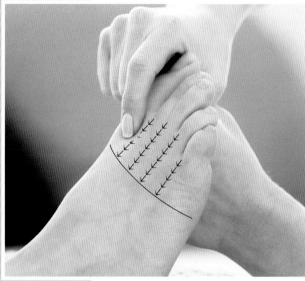

10 Breast and lung (plantar)
Hold the right foot with your left hand. Using your right thumb, creep up to the areas between the grooves of each toe on the sole of the foot as shown. Change hands to treat the left foot.

11 Breast and lung (dorsal)
Press your left fist into the sole of the right foot. Creep down from the grooves below the toes on the top of the foot with your right index finger as shown. Change hands to work the left foot.

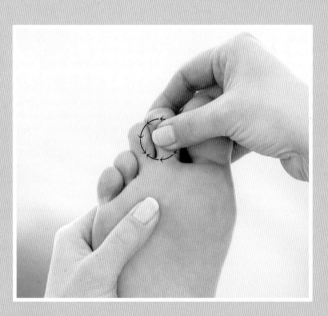

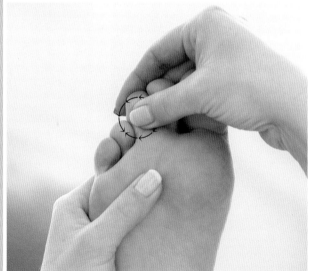

12 Eye
Hold the right foot with your left hand. Placing your right thumb just below the first bend of the second toe and make a small rotating movement to work the reflex. Change hands to work the left foot.

13 Ear
Hold the right foot with your left hand. Placing your right thumb just under the first bend of the third toe and work the reflex with a small rotating movement. Change hands to work the left foot.

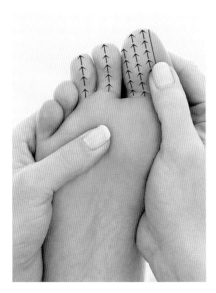

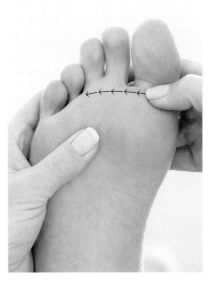

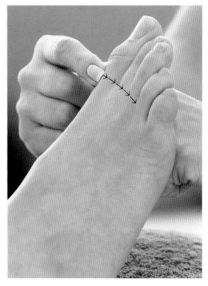

14 Sinuses

Hold the right foot with your left hand. With your right thumb, creep up each of the first three toes. Switch hands and work back. Work the left foot starting with your right hand.

15 Neck and thyroid (plantar)

Holding the right foot with your left hand, creep across the base of the first three toes three times. Change hands to work the left foot.

16 Neck and thyroid (dorsal)

Holding the right foot with your left fist, creep across the base of the first three toes on the top of the foot three times. Change hands to work the left foot.

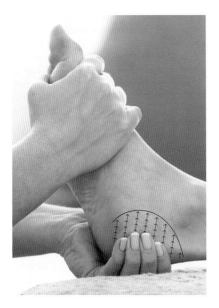

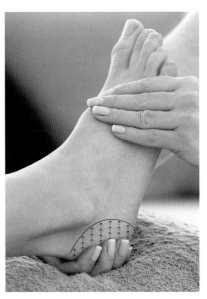

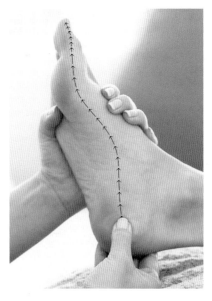

17 Coccyx

Supporting the top of the right foot with your right hand, creep up the medial side of the heel with the four fingers of your left hand. Change hands to work the left foot.

18 Hip and pelvis

Supporting the top of the right foot with your left hand, creep up the lateral side of the heel with the four fingers of your right hand. Change hands to work the left foot.

19 Spine (up)

Hold the right foot with your left hand. Creep up the inside edge of the foot to the top of the big toe with your right thumb. Change hands to work the left foot.

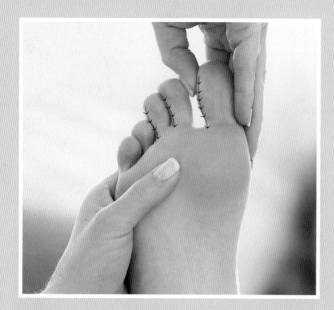

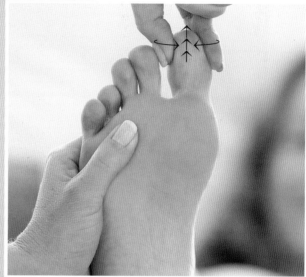

20 Chronic neck

This treatment helps all chronic neck conditions, especially in older people. Hold the right foot with your left hand. Work down the lateral sides of the first three toes with your right thumb, starting with the big toe. Change hands to work the left foot.

21 Neck rotation

The neck rotation technique will help a stiff neck in anyone suffering arthritis or whiplash injury. Hold the right foot with your left hand. Gently lift and rotate each of the first three toes in turn with your right thumb and index finger. Change hands to work the left foot.

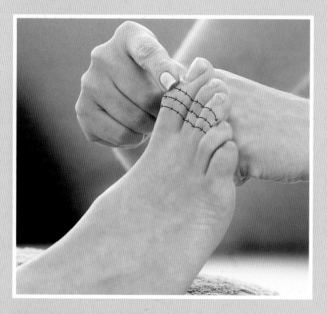

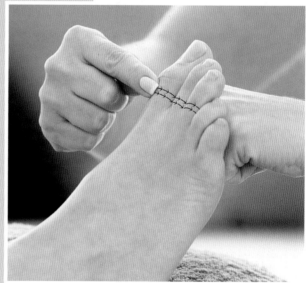

22 Face

Push your left fist into the sole of the right foot. Creep along the first three toes with your right index finger. Change hands to work the left foot.

23 Teeth

Push your left fist into the sole of the right foot. To treat the upper jaw, work across the first three toes in line with the bases of the nails with your right index finger. To treat the lower jaw, work along the first three toes just above where they join the foot. Change hands for the left foot.

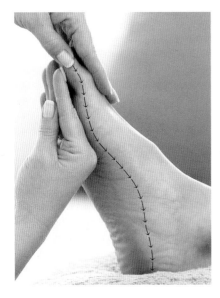

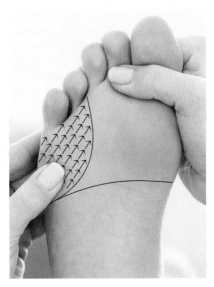

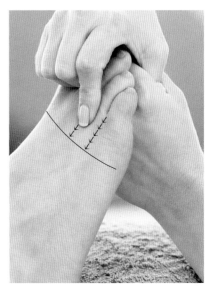

24 Spine (down)

Place the back of your right hand against the sole of the right foot. Creep down the medial edge of the foot with your left thumb. Change hands to work the left foot.

25 Shoulder (plantar)

Use your left thumb to creep upwards across the shoulder reflex area. Change hands and creep back again with your right thumb. Change hands to work the left foot.

26 Shoulder (dorsal)

Push your left fist against the sole of the right foot. Work down the grooves of the fourth and fifth toes with your right index finger. Change hands to work the left foot.

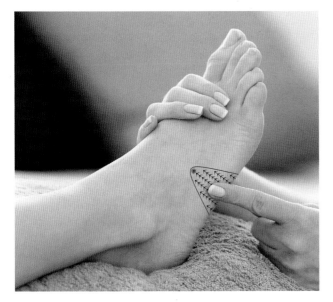

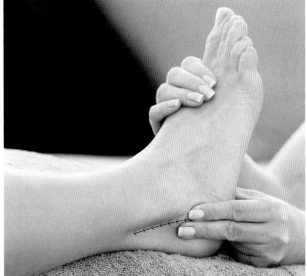

27 Knee and elbow

Hold the right foot with your left hand. Creep your right index finger up the triangular-shaped reflex on the lateral side of the foot. Change hands to work the left foot.

28 Primary sciatic

Hold the top of the right foot with your right hand. Creep your left index finger up the area behind the ankle bone, continuing about 4 cm (1½ in) up the leg. Change hands to work the left foot.

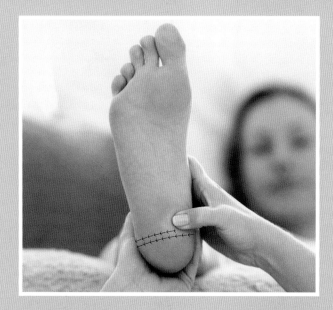

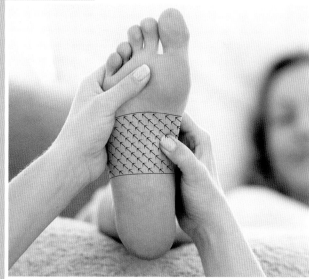

29 Secondary sciatic

Hold the right foot with your left hand. Creep your right thumb across the heel, halfway between the pelvic line (see page 10) and the bottom of the foot. Repeat two or three times, working from the medial to the lateral side. Change hands to work the left foot.

30 Liver

A good treatment for hormonal problems as the liver gets rid of excess hormones. The liver reflex is on the right foot only. Hold the foot with your left hand. Creep your right thumb across, working from the medial to the lateral side. Change hands and work back with your left thumb.

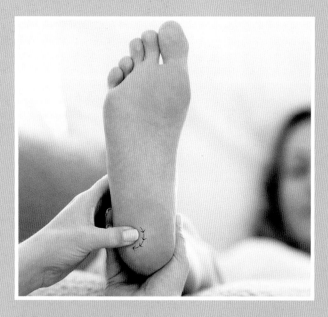

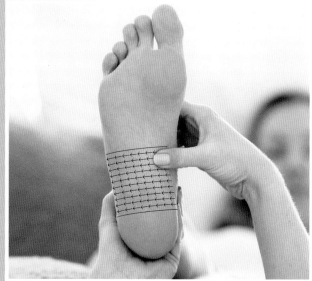

31 Ileocecal valve

This reflex is only on the right foot. Hold the foot with your right hand. Find the reflex, which lies below the pelvic line (see page 10) on the lateral side of the foot, and work with your left thumb using the hooking-out technique (see page 13).

32 Intestines

Support the right foot with your left hand. Using your right thumb, work over the area below the waist line with your right thumb, moving in straight lines from the medial to the lateral side. Change hands and use your left thumb to work back. Change hands to work the left foot.

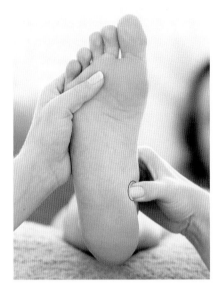

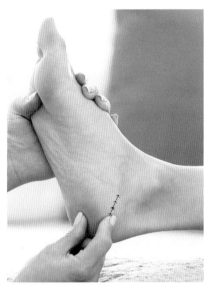

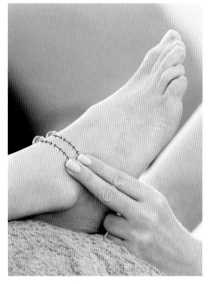

33 Bladder

Support the right foot with your left hand. Work over the bladder reflex – the soft area on the medial side – two or three times with your right thumb. Change hands for the left foot.

34 Uterus

Hold the right foot with your left hand. With your right index finger, work from the tip of the heel to the ankle bone on the medial side of the foot. Change hands for the left foot.

35 Fallopian tubes

Hold the foot, pressing into the sole with both thumbs. Using the index and third fingers of both hands, creep across the top of the foot two or three times.

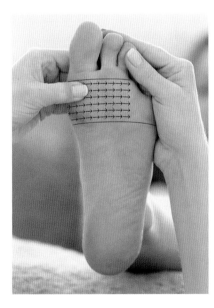

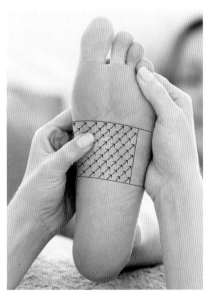

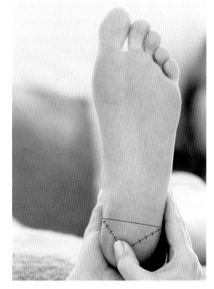

36 Heart

The main heart reflex is on the left foot, beneath the first three toes. Hold the foot with your right hand and creep across from the big toe to the third toe with your left thumb.

37 Stomach and pancreas

The main reflex for the stomach is on the left foot. Work over the area with your left thumb, moving from the medial to the lateral side. Work back across the area with your right thumb.

38 Sigmoid colon

This V-shaped reflex is found only on the left foot. With your right thumb, creep up the outside fork of the reflex area. Change hands and creep up the inside fork with your right thumb.

Index

Further reading

Ann Gillanders has written a number of other books on reflexology. These include the following:

Reflexology: A step-by-step Guide
Gaia Books, 1995

The Family Guide to Reflexology
Gaia Books, 1998

Reflexology: A Busy Person's Guide
Gaia Books, 2002

Reflexology for Back Pain
Gaia Books, 2005

ANN GILLANDERS REFLEXOLOGY INTERNATIONAL PUBLICATIONS, AVAILABLE FROM REFLEXOLOGY SALES Tel. 01279 429060: www.footreflexology.com

Gateways to Health and Harmony, 1987

Reflexology: The Ancient Answer to Modern Ailments, 1987

No Mean Feat (autobiography), 1990

Reflexology – The Theory and Practice, 1994

The Essential Guide to Foot and Hand Reflexology, 1998

Reflexology and the Intestinal Link, 1999

The Compendium of Healing Points, 2001

For more information on reflexology, contact Ann Gillanders Reflexology International, incorporating The British School of Reflexology,
92 Sheering Road
Old Harlow
Essex CM17 0JW

Tel: 01279 429060
Fax: 01279 445234
ann@footreflexology.com
www:footreflexology.com

Useful addresses

ACTIVE BIRTH CENTRE
Bickerton House, 25 Bickerton Road
London N19 5JT
Tel: 020 7281 6790
www.activebirthcentre.com
Email: info@activebirthcentre.com

AIMS (Association for Improvements in
Maternity Services)
5 Ann's Court, Grove Road, Surbiton, Surrey KT6 4BE
Tel: 0870 765 1433
www.aims.org.uk

FORESIGHT ASSOCIATION FOR THE PROMOTION
OF PRECONCEPTUAL CARE
178 Hawthorn Road, West Bognor
West Sussex PO21 2UY
Tel: 01243 868001
Fax: 01243 868180
www.foresight-preconception.org.uk

NATIONAL CHILDBIRTH TRUST
Alexandra House
Oldham Terrace
London W3 6NH
Tel: 0870 770 3236
www.nctpregnancyandbabycare.com
Emails: enquiries@national-childbirh-trust.co.uk

WOMEN'S HEALTH CONCERN
10 Storey's Gate
London SW1P 3AY
Tel: 020 7799 9897
www.womens-health-concern.org

WOMEN'S HEALTH
52 Featherstone Street
London EC1Y 8RT
Tel: 020 7251 6333
www.womenshealthlondon.org.uk
Email: info@womenshealthlondon.org.uk

Acknowledgements

Author's acknowledgements.

I would like to express my appreciation to Jinny for her expertise and professional support in editing this book. And to Phil Gamble for his artistic design skills and photographic excellence, it was a great joy to work with them both.

Editor Jinny Johnson
Co-ordination Camilla Davis
Direction Jo Godfrey Wood, Leigh Jones
Medical consultant Dr Michael Apple
Photography Ruth Jenkinson
Production Louise Hall

Publisher's acknowledgements

Gaia Books would like to thank Constance Novis for proofreading, Elizabeth Wiggans for indexing, and Suzi Langhorne and Karen Davis for modelling for the reflexology photographs.

Photo credits
All photography Ruth Jenkinson, except the following:
1, 9, 11 Dominic Blackmore,
25, 96, 105 Gus Filgate,
55, 91 Image Source,
20, 23, 26, 38, 41, 48, 51, 53, 56, 62, 64, 71, 72, 79, 80, 87, 88, 109, 113 Corbis.